A JOURNEY INTO
Health Qigong

The Chinese Health Qigong Association (CHQA) is a group member of All-China Sports Federation, the only national qigong community organization in China. Headquartered in Beijing, CHQA has devoted itself to the exploration and dissemination of the essence of traditional qigong culture and health qigong exercises for the benefit of the physical and mental health of humankind.

In recent years, CHQA has compiled 9 sets of exercises, including *Yi Jin Jin, Wu Qin Xi, Liu Zi Jue,* and *Ba Duan Jin*, all of which are based on traditional qigong practices. Due to popular demand, CHQA will revive more qigong forms to be taught to the public.

Project Editors: Zeng Chun, Mei Li & Liu Shui
Copy Editor: Li Wang-ling (Phoenix Li)
Book Designer: Li Xi
Cover Designer: Li Xi
Typesetter: He Mei ling

A JOURNEY INTO
Health Qigong
Chinese Health Qigong Association

Editor-in-Chief
Xiao Min
Vice-Chairman, Chinese Olympic Committee, Beijing, China

Associate Editors-in-Chief
Ji Yun-xi
Vice-Chairman, Chinese Health Qigong Association, Beijing, China

Zou Ji-jun
Vice-Chairman, Chinese Health Qigong Association, Beijing, China

Translators
Li Wang-ling (Phoenix Li) & **Wang Jun-fa**

English Language Editor
Dane Dormio (USA)

PMPH PEOPLE'S MEDICAL PUBLISHING HOUSE

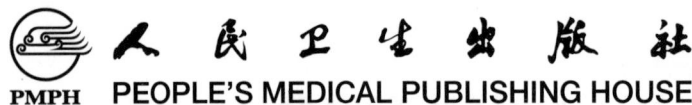
PEOPLE'S MEDICAL PUBLISHING HOUSE

Website: http://www.pmph.com

Book Title: A Journey Into Health Qigong
走进健身气功

Copyright © 2010 by People's Medical Publishing House. All rights reserved. No part of this publication may be reproduced, stored in a database or retrieval system, or transmitted in any form or by any electronic, mechanical, photocopy, or other recording means, without the prior written permission of the publisher.

Contact address: No. 19, Pan Jia Yuan Nan Li, Chaoyang District, Beijing 100021, P.R. China, phone/fax: 8610 5978 7338, E-mail: pmph@pmph.com

For text and trade sales, as well as review copy enquiries, please contact PMPH at pmphsales@gmail.com

---

Disclaimer

This book is for educational and reference purposes only. In view of the possibility of human error or changes in medical science, the author, editor, publisher and any other party involved in the publication of this work do not guarantee that the information contained herein is in any respect accurate or complete. The medicinal therapies and treatment techniques presented in this book are provided for the purpose of reference only. If readers wish to attempt any of the techniques or utilize any of the medicinal therapies contained in this book, the publisher assumes no responsibility for any such actions. It is the responsibility of the readers to understand and adhere to local laws and regulations concerning the practice of these techniques and methods. The authors, editors and publishers disclaim all responsibility for any liability, loss, injury, or damage incurred as a consequence, directly or indirectly, of the use and application of any of the contents of this book.

First published: 2010
ISBN: 978 - 7 - 117 - 13623 - 5/R • 13624

Cataloguing in Publication Data:
A catalogue record for this book is available from the CIP-Database China.

Printed in The People's Republic of China

Editorial Board

Editor-in-Chief
Xiao Min
Vice-Chairman, Chinese Olympic Committee

Associate Editors-in-Chief
Ji Yun-xi
Vice-Chairman, Chinese Health Qigong Association
Zou Ji-jun
Vice-Chairman, Chinese Health Qigong Association

Contributors
Tao Zu-lai
Research Fellow, Institute of Mechanics, Chinese Academy of Sciences
Zhou Li-shang
Senior Editor, People's Sports Publishing House
Guo Shan-ru
Professor, TianJin Institute of Technology
Song Tian-bin
Professor, Beijing University of Chinese Medicine
Sun Fu-li
Research fellow, Xiyuan Hospital of China Academy of Chinese Medical Sciences
Ding Dong
Deputy Secretary-General, Chinese Health Qigong Association
Zhu Ying
Member, Standing Committee of Chinese Health Qigong Association
Cui Yong-sheng
Dr., Assistant Research Fellow, Health Qigong Management Center, China General Administration of Sports

Editor's Note

For the dedicated qigong practitioner, this book is a valuable gem indeed. The information it provides can accelerate the journey of our practice in at least four ways:

- It gives specific guidelines for getting the most benefit from practice. All practitioners of qigong can benefit from taking these precepts to heart.

- It provides conceptual tools, important for approaching and thinking about our qigong practice with an appropriate understanding and attitude.

- One of the precepts of qigong practice is "Improve Theoretical Understanding and Cultivate Scientific Awareness". Studying this book goes towards fulfilling this precept.

- Certainly not least in importance, this book provides an abundance of inspiration to practice by delivering loudly and clearly the good news that we can all use the power of our minds and self-directed exercise to overcome illness and generate good health, as recorded since ancient times and confirmed by modern science, helping to spark off a virtuous cycle of health preservation!

Do not let the value that this book can provide go to waste. Read it, certainly, but don't stop there. Internalize it in your practice (start practicing if you don't already) and embody it in your daily life. Then, share the knowledge you have gained. Encourage others to read it and join you in your practice.

Here's to a healthier, happier, more beautiful world.

Dane Dormio
San Diego, CA, USA
September 2010

Translator's Note

It has been my great pleasure to work on the English version of "A Journey into Health Qigong", produced by the Chinese Health Qigong Association. It has been both a challenging and interesting project, since this is the first book on the theoretical foundation of health qigong to be published in English, and many of the terms and quotes have never been translated before.

It is never easy to translate intangible concepts, especially the ancient terms and quotes which have appeared frequently in this book. In classical Chinese, each character conveys an extensive meaning, and the meaning varies depending on how and where it is being used, making it impossible to assign a fixed English term to represent it. Often the best thing to do then is to adopt the use of the word directly into English using a Romanization such as *pinyin*, as we have already accepted with words like yin, yang, tai ji, and qigong. This is what was done with some of the ambiguous terms in this book. Also, I've added as many notes as possible to explain potentially confusing concepts, in the hope of making them more understandable to you, the reader.

There will never be enough time to create a perfect translation, especially when sophisticated theories are involved. Projects must be completed in haste, however, and I can only wish to have more time to spend improving it. As a health qigong practitioner myself, I have a strong affection for this project and I hope that we not only bring you an enjoyable reading experience but also help you find the motivation to start practicing and experiencing health qigong.

I would like to acknowledge my gratitude for the help of a few persons: my editor, Dane Dormio, for making this book a more readable and enjoyable one; Jane Zeng and others from PMPH for all their support and understanding; Douglas Eisenstark in Los Angeles for all the advice and inspiration he gave to me in this project; and finally Zhang Ming-liang, who is one of the writers of the Chinese version of this book as well as my mentor in both qigong and traditional Chinese medicine.

Li Wan-ling (Phoenix Li)
Beijing, China
September, 2010

Preface

Health qigong is a traditional national sport. Its main form of exercise is a combination of physical activities that cater to the needs of breathing and psychological adjustment. It is a key component of Chinese culture and has been popular for thousands of years, owing to its health benefits and ease of practice. Its gentle, soft, and slow movements make it suitable for young and old alike.

In recent years, the popularity of health qigong has grown. With its diverse expressions and unique charm, health qigong has captured the attention of practitioners from across China and the globe. It has become a picturesque part of the landscape of Chinese national fitness.

As health qigong has become more publicly known, curiosity has grown. More people want to know about its unique features, what it is and how it is different from other types of qigong, as well as about its benefits and best methods of practice.

Theory guides action. Mastering scientific concepts and methods of fitness can not only foster health and happiness for the individual, but also promote the harmony and progress of society. Conversely, lacking a scientific understanding can cause confusion. Learning about the underlying theory is central to benefiting from health qigong. Promoting the scientific concepts inherent to this form of exercise beautifully upholds the ideology of qigong practice.

This book is intended to help the reader understand what health qigong is all about using non-technical terminology. Its chapters fall into three main sections. Chapters 1, 2, and 3 provide an overview of the world health situation and how health qigong fits into it, and also lay the conceptual groundwork necessary for understanding health qigong. They make a good, quick introduction to the subject for beginners. Chapters 4 and 5 introduce four health qigong routines and outline their features and benefits. Chapters 6, 7, 8, and 9 detail the scientifically documented health benefits of health qigong and provide a thorough guideline for progressing in one's own practice.

Chinese Health Qigong Association
Beijing, China
September, 2010

Contents

Chapter 1 General Overview 1
    Health, Sub-health, and Disease 1
        Definition of Health 1
        Health and Disease 2
        Definition of Sub-health 3
        Sub-health and Disease 4
        Senility and Life Expectancy 4
    The Importance of Health Exercises 5
        Nipping Disease in the Bud 6
        Approaching Health Exercises Systematically 6
        Myths of Health Exercises 7

Chapter 2 Understanding Health Qigong 8
    History of Health Qigong 8
        Origin of Qigong 8
        Development of Qigong 9
        Concepts of Health Qigong 12
    Key Elements of Health Qigong Practice 13
        Body Regulation 13
        Breath Regulation 14
        Mind Regulation 16

Chapter 3 Health Qigong Concepts 18
    Health Qigong & Health Cultivation 18
        Traditional Chinese Health Cultivation 18
        Qigong Health Cultivation 18
        Dietary Health Cultivation 19
        Medical Health Cultivation 19
        Health Cultivation According to the Four Seasons 20
        Health Cultivation in Daily Life 21

  Health Cultivation through Leisure Activities 21
 Health Qigong as the Critical Component of TCHC 22
  For Improving Physical Condition 22
  For Disease Prevention 23
  For Resisting Senility and Prolonging Life 23
  For Mental Regulation and Cultivating Morals 24
 Principles of Health Cultivation Applied in Health Qigong 24
  Body Regulation 24
  Breath Regulation 25
  Mind Regulation 27

Chapter 4 Introduction to Health Qigong Routines 29
 The Four Health Qigong Routines 29
  Health Qigong *Yi Jin Jing* 29
  Health Qigong *Wu Qin Xi* 32
  Health Qigong *Liu Zi Jue* 34
  Health Qigong *Ba Duan Jin* 35
 Principles Guiding the Creation of Health Qigong Routines 37
  Principles of Strengthening the Body and Cultivating Health 37
  Using Science as a Yardstick in the Development of Health Qigong 38

Chapter 5 Features of Health Qigong 40
 Health Qigong Qualifies as Aerobic Exercise 40
 Health Qigong Emphasizes the Overall Training of Body and Mind 41
 Health Qigong is Target-Oriented, Safe and Reliable 42
 Health Qigong is Easy to Practice 43
 Health Qigong Inherits the Best of Tradition and Modern Times 43
  Health Qigong Draws upon the Quintessence of Tradition 44
  Health Qigong Meets the Needs of Modern Times 44
  Health Qigong Incorporates Collective Wisdom to
   Withstand the Test of History 45

Chapter 6 Physiological Effects of Health Qigong 46
 General Effects 46
  Effects on the Nervous System 47
  Effects on the Endocrine System 47

- Effects on the Cardiovascular System 48
- Effects on the Digestive System 48
- Effects on Hematopoiesis (The Formation of Blood) 49
- Effects on the Immune System 49
- **Specific Benefits** 50
  - Regulating Heart Rate and Blood Pressure 50
  - Improving Blood Supply to the Heart 50
  - Reversing Cardio- and Cerebrovascular Disease 51
  - Improving Lung Capacity 51
  - Slowing Aging 52

Chapter 7 Health Qigong and Psychological Health 54
- **Health Qigong and Cognitive Ability** 54
  - Preventing Intelligence Decline 54
  - Improving Attention 55
  - Promoting Imagination 56
- **Health Qigong and Mood Regulation** 56
  - The Influence of Emotions on Health 56
  - The Influence of Health Qigong Practice on Mood 57
  - Psychological Explanation for Health Qigong's Effect on Mood 58
- **Health Qigong and the Optimization of Personality** 58
  - Cultivation of Morals 59
  - Effects on Type A Personality 59
- **Health Qigong and Interpersonal Relationships** 60
  - Interpersonal Relationships and Mental and Physical Health 60
  - Factors Affecting Interpersonal Relationships 61
  - Health Qigong's Influence on Interpersonal Relationships 61
  - Health Qigong as a Platform for Communication 62
- **Health Qigong and a Healthy Lifestyle** 62
  - The Importance of a Healthy Lifestyle 63
  - Health Qigong's Effects on Lifestyle 63
- **Health Qigong as Part of a Healthy Lifestyle** 64
- **Health Qigong as a Bridge to a Healthy Lifestyle** 65
  - Health Qigong Can Help in Quitting Unhealthy Habits 65
  - Health Qigong as a Way of Learning about Health Cultivation 65
  - Health Qigong Leads to Psychological Balance 66

Health Qigong Induces a Harmonious Society.. 66

Chapter 8 Principles of Health Qigong Practice... 68
Laying a Solid Mental Foundation 68
Confidence 68
Determination.. 68
Perseverance 69
Contented Heart 69
Principles of Health Qigong Practice.. 70
Unification of Body, Mind, and Qi 70
Relaxation and Tranquility 70
Motion (Dynamic) and Stillness (Static) 72
Obeying the Laws of Nature 73
Obeying the Laws of Nature in Health Qigong Practice 73
Obeying the Laws of Nature in Health Cultivation 74
Obeying the Laws of Nature to Preserve Vitality.............................. 74
Relaxation as a Principle of Nature 74
Combining Health Qigong and Health Cultivation 75
About Health Cultivation.. 75
Health Qigong and a Healthy Lifestyle... 76

Chapter 9 Precepts of Health Qigong Practice... 78
Discard Mental Burdens.. 78
Relax Body and Mind Completely.. 78
Proceed Gradually... 78
Inject Perseverance throughout Practice 79
Be Intentional about Choosing Exercises 80
Subdivide the "Three Regulations" 80
Stress the Features of Each Routine 81
Practice Hard... 82
Be Mindful of the Warming Up and Closing Movements................ 83
Improve Theoretical Understanding and Cultivate Scientific Awareness....... 83
Create Good Conditions for Practice... 84

Chapter 10 The Scientific Approach to Health Qigong Practice 85
Techniques for Health Qigong *Yi Jin Jing* 85

Proper Application of Strength 85
Natural Breathing 86
Concentration of the Mind 87
The Opening and Closing Posture of Health Qigong *Wu Qin Xi* 88
Ready Position: Adjusting the Breath 88
Difficult Points in the Opening Posture 89
Common Mistakes in the Opening Posture 90
The "Three Regulations" in the Opening Posture 90
Closing Posture: Convey Qi to *Dantian* 91
Keys and Techniques in Health Qigong *Liu Zi Jue* 92
Correct Pronunciation 92
How to Pronounce the Sounds in *Liu Zi Jue* 93
The Volume of Sound 93
Mouth Shape and Tips for the Breathing Technique 93
About "Breath" 98
The Keys for Learning and Practicing Health Qigong *Ba Duan Jin* 98
Health Qigong *Ba Duan Jin* Focuses on the Training of the Body 98
The Exercise of the Spine is the Core of Health Qigong *Ba Duan Jin* 99
The "Ready Position" is Critical in Health Qigong *Ba Duan Jin* 103

Chapter 11 Notes for Health Qigong Practice 105
Grasping the Scientific Approach 105
The Purpose of Practice 105
Preparation before Practice 106
Paying Attention to the Movements 106
Practice according to Your Own Condition 107
Effects Determined by Details 107

Chapter 12 Issues in Health Qigong Practice 109
Motion and Stillness 109
The Differentiation and Unity of "Motion" and "Stillness" 109
"Stillness" within "Motion" 109
"Motion" Manifested through "Stillness" 110
"Relaxation" and "Tension" 111
Application of "Relaxation" and "Tension" 111
"Relaxation" and "Tension" in Body Movements 111

    The "Relaxation" and "Tension" of the Mind 113
"Stirring Sensations" 114
    The Concept of "Stirring Sensations" 114
    How to Overcome "Stirring Sensations" 114
    Problems Caused by Improper Practice 115
Group Practice and Individual Practice 115
    Benefits of Group Practice 115
    Benefits of Individual Practice 116
    Integrating Group Practice and Individual Practice 116
    Practice Where a Certified Health Qigong Tutor is Available 117
Practicing a Single Routine or Practicing All the Routines Together 117
    Body Movements in Common 117
    Qi and Blood Circulation and Breathing Techniques in Common 118
    Proficiency with a Single Routine or with All Routines 119

Chapter 13 Health Qigong Testimonials 120

Appendix Major Acupoints of the Human Body 126

Afterword 141

Index 143

Chapter 1

General Overview

Health, Sub-health, and Disease

Definition of Health

Health is the first form of wealth. Without health, money cannot be enjoyed, and dreams cannot be realized regardless of aggressiveness or capability. Without health, lasting happiness and quality of life are impossible to achieve.

Health is also the wealth of a society. In 2001, China's total consumption of health care resources cost 614 billion Chinese Yuan (RMB), accounting for 6.4% of the GDP. The sum of financial losses resulting from disease, disability, and premature death was 780 billion RMB, or 8.2% of the GDP. The combined cost of these was 1.4 trillion RMB, or 14.6% of the GDP. What should be troubling is that in recent years the growth rate of this figure has exceeded the growth rate of the national economy and per capita income. For the sake of comparison to the 1.4 trillion RMB spent on health-related costs in 2001, the total cost of the famous Three Gorges 15-year project is only 200 billion RMB; the total cost of the South-North Water Diversion 50-year Project is only 500 billion RMB. Both of these figures are dwarfed by the amount spent on health-related costs in a single year. More importantly, health problems exacerbate poverty and cause immeasurable physical and mental pain. The growing medical problem has thus become a hot spot of society as well as a focus of government policies. It should be a vexing issue for other governments around the globe as well.

The definition of health given by the World Health Organization (WHO) is: "A state of complete physical, mental, and social wellbeing, and not merely the absence of disease or infirmity."

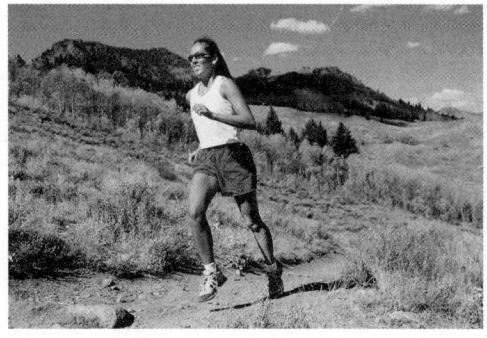

Some of the physical attributes associated with good health are the following: body systems are operating normally, weight and body shape are appropriate, eyes are bright and sharp, eyelids are without inflammation, teeth are clean and without defects or pain or bleeding of the gums, hair is thick and without dandruff, muscles are flexible and skin is elastic, the step is light while walking, energy is steady throughout the day while sleep is sound at night, resistance to illness and infection is strong, and the person is adaptable to different environments.

Good health also encompasses the personality: stable emotions, a moderate character, a strong will with rich feelings, an open mind, an active, optimistic attitude, a willingness to bear responsibilities, and a generous heart.

A healthy personality bestows a strong ability to deal with anything that comes, to be objective and realistic while observing problems, to maintain self discipline in the face of adversity, to deal with emergencies, and to adapt to a complex social environment. A healthy personality invokes good interpersonal relationships and is obliging, kind, and compassionate towards others.

Good health requires positive habits, including a regular schedule. This means not only making good use of working time, but also making adequate arrangements for rest and recreation. It is important to have meaningful work that keeps you busy but doesn't lead to overly stressed states or chaos, as well as sufficient leisure and relaxation. Good health habits also include not harming yourself by overindulging in pleasures, but rather implementing the discipline of moderation.

Health and Disease

Health is a difficult concept to measure objectively. A person can only be considered healthy if certain elements of wellbeing exist, but absolute health must be an ideal that can never be truly achieved. The WHO's definition of "health" has captured this property.

For a long time it was held that health is a state without disease, but this view is very limiting because it inevitably leaves a gap for disease to foster. A more beneficial concept of health is a state of happiness and enjoyment of life. This view both provides direction for growth and makes good health easier to assess, thus the Chinese saying: "Health is like water in a well: the importance of the water can never be realized until the well is dry."

A tendency many people have is to magnify whatever disease may be present in their body by feeding it with anxiety and worry. People who panic upon hearing bad news about their health often make the situation worse, or even create an illness where none existed to begin with.

Other people tend to live in a fantastic inner world, but never face reality on its own terms. These people may have strong ambitions to create a beautiful life but lack the courage to bring them to fruition. This type of person may go through a physical examination and find nothing wrong with their body, and thus be incorrectly labeled "healthy", but actually they may be in poor psychological health. Health needs to be measured by how a person feels and performs as well as by how well their physical body functions.

Moderation is one powerful key to living a happy life. Too much of anything can be destructive. Thus, maintaining optimum health demands responsibility in the form of being able to objectively see and consciously separate the passions of the body and the discipline of the mind. This form of responsibility makes it easier to make healthy, positive choices.

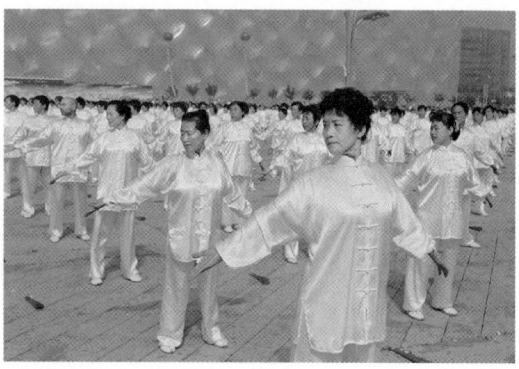

In the 21st century, people are paying more and more attention to their own health, and the focus of their attention is shifting from medical treatment to disease prevention. This consciousness shift is a step in the right direction. Everyone deserves to be healthy. Maintaining and increasing health requires a new perception of health as alive and ever-changing. This attitude makes it easier to respond to the requirements of maintaining good health. The pursuit of medicine in the 21st century is not about treating illness better, but about helping people (especially the elderly) lead healthier lives.

Definition of Sub-health

As medical knowledge has progressed, a new concept has emerged called "sub-health" that transcends previously existing concepts of wellness and disease. Sub-health is an intermediate state of the human being between health and illness. This concept is accommodated by the WHO's definition of health, which acknowledges that health is more than the lack of disease. The state of sub-health is also known as the "premorbid state", or the "preclinical period". A state of sub-health is indicated by "three declines" (declines of energy, responsiveness, and adaptability), "three highs and one low" (hyperlipidemia, hyperglycemia, high blood viscosity, and low immunity), and "syndromes of five diseases" (obesity, hypertension, coronary heart disease, diabetes, and stroke). A global survey by the WHO concluded that while healthy people make up 5% of the population and diseased people make up 20%, the rest of us, 75%, are sub-healthy. The number of sub-healthy people is growing in many countries, and the phenomenon is becoming a hotspot of research by the international medical community.

Sub-health is very complex because it involves many aspects of a person's life, including physiology, psychology, and society. These are some common experiences associated with sub-health conditions: physical fatigue, vulnerability to colds and infections, tiring easily, frequent perspiring or cold sweating, rough skin, fast heartbeat, irregular blood pressure, poor appetite, insomnia, jittery mood, irritability, lack of focus, nervousness and anxiety, social fatigue, discord and disharmony within personal and family relationships, and sexual disorders. Many times sub-health may manifest as an inexpressible sense of discomfort that doesn't show up on any examination results. Generally speaking, the state of feeling sick or unwell without having a disease is sub-health.

Fortunately, sub-health has a simple cause and a simple remedy: diet and lifestyle habits. To use the situation in China as an example, many of the health challenges found in China revolve around diet. As China modernizes it adopts more and more a typical Western diet, with high fat and cholesterol content and unbalanced nutrition. Over time, such a diet leads to the diseases of civilization characterized by the "three highs" (hypertension, hyperglycemia, and hyperlipidemia), especially among middle-aged and older people. Furthermore, the more time people spend in work settings as opposed to natural settings, the more their exercise habits tend to suffer. According to studies, the number of sub-healthy people in China exceeds 0.7 billion, accounting for 60% to 70% of the population. A study of 16 Chinese metropolitan areas concluded that the highest rate of sub-health is in Beijing, at 75.31%, closely followed by Shanghai and Guangdong, which are at 73.49% and 73.41%, respectively.

Sub-health and Disease

Sub-health itself is not a disease, but it coincides with the process of cumulative and gradual changes that often take place before a disease breaks out. A person in a state of sub-health may be moving in either direction, moving into either better or worse health.

Other research indicates that 48% of workers within 10 major cities in China are considered to be in a state of sub-health. The percentage is generally higher in coastal cities and less so in inland cities. Also, the rate tends to be higher among employees who do mostly "brain" work as compared with employees who do more physical work, and higher among middle-aged people than among younger people. From these results, it is obvious that sub-health is an invisible "killer" hiding in our body, a "chronic suicide" leading us to diseases and ultimately death. Therefore, we should not ignore even the slightest signs of sub-health within our body.

The importance of being aware of the condition of sub-health as a scale can't be overestimated. It can provide guidance for individuals and groups to make health-related decisions, including when to seek professional help.

Senility and Life Expectancy

The growth of the human body peaks at a typical age of about 25, after which point the body starts to age. Aging is a long but slow process.

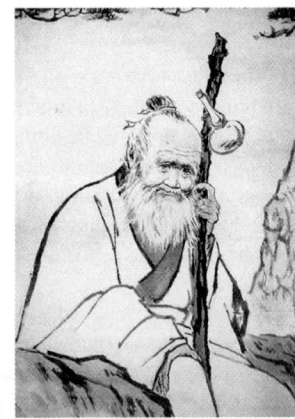

From a biological perspective, the human body is capable of living about 120 years. So, why is it that we seldom hear of people who live to be this age? This can largely be attributed to poor lifestyle habits. There are many factors which can influence lifespan and the speed of aging, and our body will automatically react to these factors which prevent us from living a purely natural life. An obvious factor is disasters, whether natural or artificial, but many diseases can also shorten life by accelerating the aging process. Even after recovering from a serious disease or damage, the body may not be able to attain its former energy level.

Even common illnesses like colds and the flu can accelerate the aging process and lower the quality of life. Though such illnesses are not life-threatening, they still erode the body's resources. Thus, maintaining healthful living habits and having a strong immune system both help to increase lifespan.

In a state of sub-health, the human body is in chronic fatigue, and the mind may be in a constant state of stress and anxiety, which is often overlooked in Western medicine, but which consumes energy and accelerates aging. Theoretically, the total number of heartbeats in a person's lifetime is fixed at about 2.5 to 3 billion. If a person's heart often palpitates, as with tachycardia, it could be said that they are aging faster and shortening their lifespan.

Disasters, major diseases, minor illnesses, and the state of sub-health are all detrimental to both the quality and length of life, and efforts made to minimize them will probably pay off in a happier, longer life for any individual.

The Importance of Health Exercises

Worldwide, the economic burdens imposed by disease and sub-health are trending upward. More and more individuals and governments in the Western developed countries are seeking the therapies of "alternative medicine", such as Traditional Chinese Medicine (TCM), qigong, and other forms of therapy that invoke mental and physical balance, to compensate for the inadequacies of mainstream Western medicine and to reduce the financial impact of disease and sub-health. The prevalence of sub-health has attracted broad attention from the medical profession. However, since sub-health is not a disease, Western medicine, which is accustomed to designing treatments in accordance with pathological diseases, is not suited to address it.

On the other hand, many so-called "alternative medical therapies", particularly TCM, qigong and physical training, are highly suited to addressing the issue of sub-health. These work outside the parameters of Western medicine, incorporating biology, psychology, and society as integral facets of the individual's wellbeing. Such healing modalities, especially when coupled with health exercises such as qigong, can improve health, prevent disease, improve the quality of life, and slow aging. As an example, a study indicates that a man who spends an hour or more per day walking has one-fourth the risk of dying from ischemic heart disease of one who seldom exercises.

Obviously, there is an important place in the world for exercises that are scientifically designed to work for anyone to increase health and heal disease, of which qigong would serve as an example. Health exercises reduce tiredness and boost adaptability and endurance, thus lowering the likelihood for disease to set in. There is an ancient principle in TCM: "curing diseases before they happen"; many of the TCM syndromes, such as the "deficiency syndromes", are believed to be manifestations of sub-health.

Treatment of sub-health conditions must be both personal and scientific. Modern treatments are moving toward "personalized medicine", according to which treatment plans are created based on the patient's individual situation, with the intention of maximizing the effects of the treatment. Moderate exercise plans, like "sports prescriptions" made by regular sports clubs, can be designed in accordance with the diversity of individual physical conditions. For example, eye exercises are important for middle and primary school students to prevent myopia, while neck and shoulder exercises are important for computer operators to strengthen cervical vertebrae. Such plans are both personalized and scientifically designed. TCM has always emphasized the variations among individuals and adapting treatments to suit the times and local conditions. Similarly, qigong exercises that are suitable for one person may not be suitable for another, so exercise routines are meant to be adapted to the individual practitioner.

Nipping Disease in the Bud

The WHO has suggested the strategy of "preventative health", which actually means reducing and preventing sub-health. The concept of prevention requires initiative. For example, taking the initiative to rest before you become tired prevents exhaustion, and drinking before you are thirsty prevents dehydration. Likewise, supplementing vitamins and trace elements before diseases or symptoms of deficiency appear is both proactive and preventive. A sick body cannot absorb or use nutrients as readily as a healthy one can.

Health exercises follow the same principle. A clever practitioner won't wait for signs of disease to appear, but rather will take the initiative to exercise in order to stay as far as possible from sub-health and disease.

Approaching Health Exercises Systematically

Health exercises should be approached from a systematic and long-term perspective that incorporates psychology and lifestyle. Without these elements, health exercises cannot achieve their greatest effect. Remember that Rome wasn't built in a day. The more closely you follow the principles and the longer you persist, the more apparent the benefits will become.

Health exercises go hand in hand with a healthy personality and a healthy lifestyle. It is important to be able to relieve work stress and appreciate the fun in life without being either over-excited or over-anxious, and to maintain a regular schedule and a balanced diet. A balanced diet means minimizing salt and sugar and eating a wide variety of fresh plants, vegetables, and aquatic foods that replenish the body's essential nutrients, vitamins, and microelements.

In the next section, we will look at several common misunderstandings related to health exercises.

Myths of Health Exercises

Health Exercises are a One-Time Cure

Just as there is no panacea that cures all diseases, there is no single way of exercising that is optimal for every person or that will provide permanent benefits. Health must be maintained by each individual. If healthful exercise and lifestyle habits are interrupted, sub-health will silently begin to creep up. But once such habits are established, they are relatively easy to maintain, because they make you feel good!

If You Take the Right Supplements You can be Healthy without Exercising

While it is true that supplements can help to strengthen a weakened body, optimal health requires adequate exercise as well as adequate nutrition. Even a body with excellent nutrition still needs exercise. Most people who feel fatigued suffer from a lack of exercise rather than inadequate nutrition. Exercise makes the body more resistant to both stress and fatigue, and improves metabolism and overall function; but what's more, without it the body's ability to use the nutritional resources available to it will be diminished.

Health exercises are good for physical and mental health as well as for social harmony and stability. So let's get moving and take an active part in the worldwide fitness craze!

Chapter 2

Understanding Health Qigong

History of Health Qigong

Origin of Qigong

Qigong is a traditional Chinese form of exercise for fitness and health with a long, rich history. Qigong intersects with other schools of philosophy, such as the Taoist practices of *tu-na*[1], *fu-qi*[2], *xing-qi*[3], *nei-dan*[4], and *cun-si*[5]; Buddhist Zen practices, meditation, and *guan-xiang*[6]; *dao-yin*[7], *an-qiao*[8]; medical diet and studies on daily lifestyle from medicine; and Confucian practices of self-cultivation, qi-cultivation and *zuo-wang*[9]. Qigong, due to its special charms such as being soft and slow and bestowing obvious health benefits to young and old, has been popular in various forms for thousands of years.

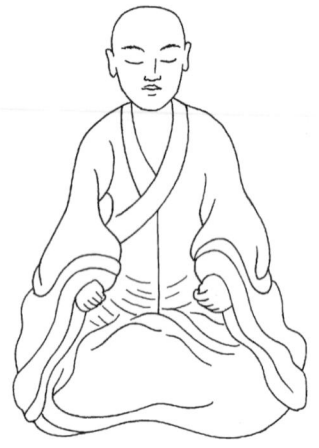

Qigong was developed from the accumulated experiences of daily life and work. Among the qigong exercises are many physical movements and breathing techniques which are the prototypes of movements from our daily life and work. As examples, consider how when we feel tired we often like to stretch out with both arms straight over our heads, which is an embryonic form of certain movements in the qigong routine *Ba Duan Jin*; or how when we are upset and exhausted we sometimes close our eyes to get a rest from vexation, which is characterized in many exercises and is known as "concentrating the mind to be tranquil".

---

1. *tu-na*: Exhalation and inhalation, a traditional term for breathing exercises.
2. *fu-qi*: Qi taking, a traditional practice of qigong.
3. *xing-qi*: Qi directing, a traditional practice of qigong.
4. *nei-dan*: Internal elixir, a traditional Taoist practice of qigong.
5. *cun-si*: Mind induction, a traditional practice (mind regulation technique) of qigong, meditation and other cultivation practices.
6. *guan-xiang*: Visualization and contemplation, a mind regulation technique in qigong, meditation, and other cultivation practices by using symbolic imagination.
7. *dao-yin*: The traditional term for health exercises or qigong practices which use the methods of body movements.
8. *an-qiao*: An ancient term for massage.
9. *zuo-wang*: Sitting transcendence, a traditional practice of meditation.

Since ancient times, observation has been the most basic and direct means of recognizing everything in nature. Observation is the root source of philosophical doctrines such as the harmony of humans and nature, the relatedness of the dynamic and the static, the reciprocal growth and decline of yin and yang, and the generation and restriction of the Five Elements. Through constant investigation and summarization of such natural phenomena as the movements of the sun, moon, and stars, the changing of the sky, earth, wind, and clouds, and the movements of birds, beasts, fish, and worms, ancient people assigned meanings to all things. This is how the rich theories and the numerous routines of health qigong were collected, after repeated verification through observation of nature.

For example, in one ancient painting, the *Daoyin Diagram*, unearthed in the Mawangdui Han Tomb of Changsha, Hunan, many of the movements recorded modeled those of animals: birds, bears, monkeys, wolves, apes, and even cockroaches. In the Eastern Jin Dynasty, Ge Hong (284 – 363 A.D.) mentioned movements such as *long-deng* (dragon stepping), *hu-yin* (tiger stretching), *xiong-jing* (bear moving), *gui-yan* (tortoise swallowing), *yan-fei* (swallow flying), *she-qu* (snake bending), *niao-shen* (bird extending), and *tu-jing* (rabbit shaking) in his *Bao Pu Zi/Teachings of Master Bao Pu* (*Bào Pǔ Zǐ*, 抱朴子). And of course, the most famous and representative qigong exercise routine is *Wu Qin Xi* (The Five Animal Frolic), created by Hua Tuo (25 – 220 A.D.) in the Eastern Han Dynasty.

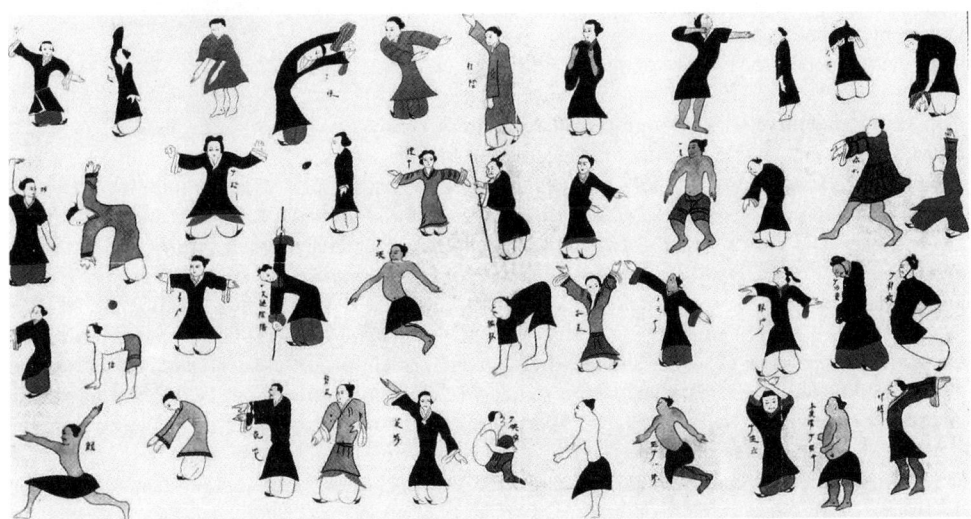

Development of Qigong

Archaeological research shows that qigong has a long history. In 1975 a relic from the Majiayao culture, a piece of colored pottery which is more than 5000 years old, was unearthed in the Ledu area

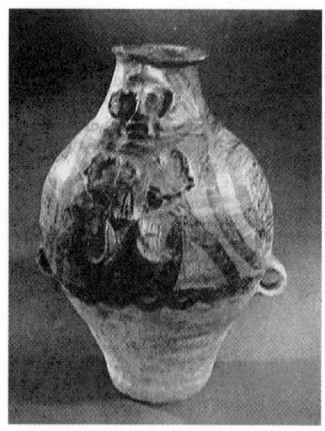

of Qinghai province. It showed a portrait of a person whose upper body was male and whose lower body was female performing breathing exercises in a standing posture. This is interpreted as showing that 5,000 years ago people were aware of the way of reconciling the yin and yang by means of breathing exercises.

Another precious cultural object related to qigong is the *The Jade Wearing with Inscription of Qi Directing* (*Xíng Qì Yù Pèi Míng*, 行气玉佩铭). The famous Chinese scientist, writer, and archaeologist, Mr. Guo Mo-ruo, interpreted the words in the inscription[10], believing that the inscription described a round of deep breathing. His interpretation is that it describes a process whereby the volume of qi is expanded with deep inhalation, then extended deeply downward and rooted firmly within the body; exhalation is the converse of inhalation, and the qi moves like a seed sprouting and growing upward. So far, historians aren't in agreement about the exact meaning of the text, but they all agree that it refers to the practice of qigong.

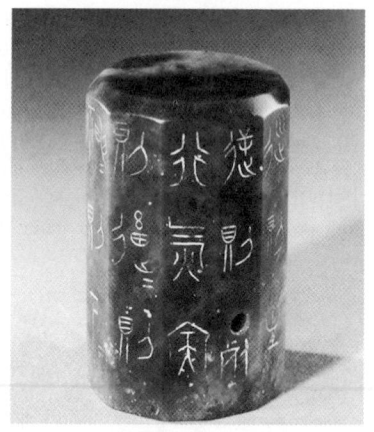

Many ancient works of literature also contain rich discussions on qigong. The practice was recorded in the *The Era of Lü – Ancient Music* (*Lǚ Shì Chūn Qiū – Gǔ Yuè*, 吕氏春秋·古乐) as follows: "*From the times of Yao Tang, yin* (*coldness and dampness*) *stagnated and accumulated within the human body; as the water ways were congested and the water could not flow freely, people mostly had constraint and stagnation diseases, their sinews and bones contracted and unable to stretch; dances were created to disperse and remove it* (*constraint and stagnation*) (昔尧唐之始，阴多滞伏而湛积，水道壅塞，不行其源，民多郁阏而滞着，筋骨瑟缩不达，故作舞以宣导之)." This text reveals that in the process of adapting to nature and the environment, ancient people created exercises (precursors of qigong) to strengthen sinews and bones, to improve circulation, to improve health, and to prevent disease.

During the Spring and Autumn Period and the Warring States Period, many schools of thought flourished. People were gaining a deeper understanding of society and nature, and they were actively studying the patterns of life, birth, growth, and death with the intent of preserving health. *The Yellow Emperor's Inner Classic* (*Huáng Dì Nèi Jīng*, 黄帝内经), written in this period, established the foundation for traditional Chinese medicine, which is the theoretical basis of qigong. The practices of *dao-yin* (body

---

10. The original Chinese text is:" 行气，深则蓄，蓄则深，深则下，下则定，定则固，固则萌，萌则长，长则退，退则天，天几　在上，地几　在下，顺则生，逆则死 "with no punctuation in between the words. There have been many debates over where the sentence should pause and the exact meaning of the words, so we did not translate it to avoid misinterpretation.

movements), *fu-qi* (qi eating), *tu-na* (exhalation and inhalation), and *xing-qi* (qi directing) have been adopted since then.

After the unification of China during the Qin Dynasty, the ruling class's pursuit of immortality encouraged the development of qigong and other health cultivation practices. Then, during the Eastern Han Dynasty, Buddhism was introduced to China along with some of its own doctrines and practices for health cultivation and the cultivation of the self. Since then, qigong has branched into three main schools: the Confucian school, the Buddhist school, and the Taoist school.

In the Three Kingdoms Period, Hua Tuo created *Wu Qin Xi* (The Five Animal Frolic), a qigong routine mimicking the movements of tigers, deer, bears, apes, and birds. This was one of the earliest qigong routines for comprehensive physical training.

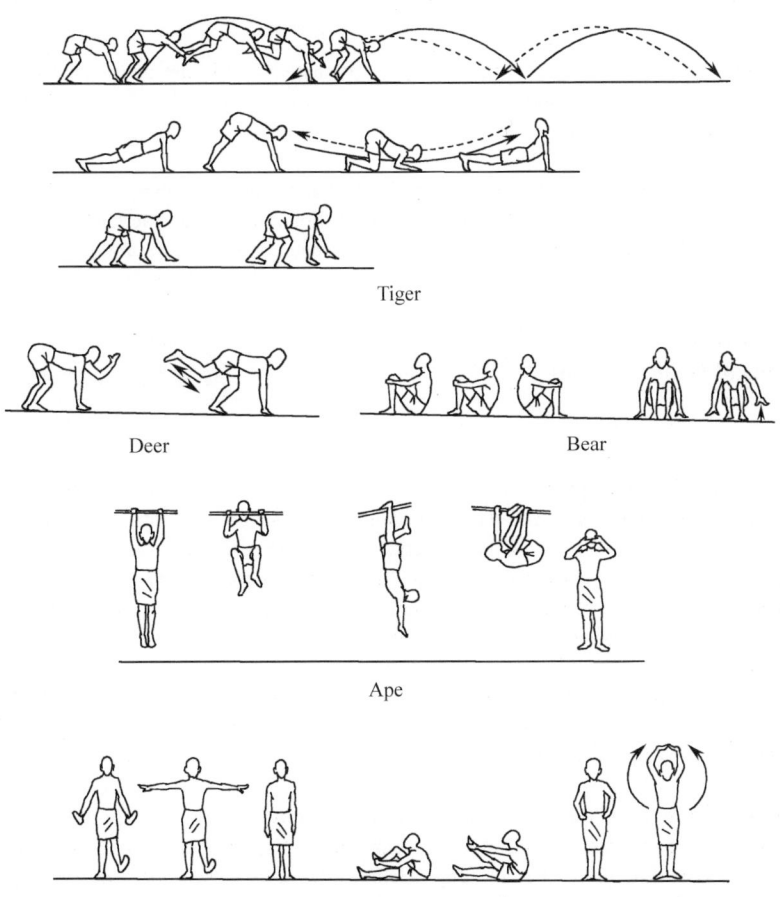

Tiger

Deer   Bear

Ape

Bird

Ge Hong's *Bao Pu Zi*, from the the Jin Dynasty, and Tao Hong-jing's *Records of Mind Cultivation and Life Prolonging* (*Yǎng Xìng Yán Mìng Lù*, 养性延命录), from the Southern and Northern Dynasties, also promoted the development of ancient qigong.

During the Sui Dynasty, the philosophies of Confucianism, Buddhism, and Taoism were applied extensively to the practice of medicine. The *Treatise on the Origins and Manifestations of Various Diseases* (*Zhū Bìng Yuán Hòu Lùn*, 诸病源候论) recorded over 260 *dao-yin* methods for promoting health and curing diseases.

During the Tang Dynasty, Sun Si-miao combined medicine, Taoism, and Buddhism in *Important Formulas Worth a Thousand Gold Pieces for Emergencies* (*Bèi Jí Qiān Jīn Yào Fāng*, 备急千金要方) and *Supplement to 'Important Formulas Worth a Thousand Gold Pieces'* (*Qiān Jīn Yì Fāng*, 千金翼方). He gave methods of "qi adjusting" and *dao-yin* that are easy to learn and particularly suitable for old people.

Throughout the Song, Yuan, Ming, and Qing dynasties, medicine developed along with the philosophies of Confucianism, Buddhism, and Taoism, forming more qigong schools and numerous new qigong routines.

Since the founding of the People's Republic of China, and especially in the past 30 years, qigong has entered a new stage of life. With tens of millions of people practicing qigong and many contributing to its development, many new routines have been built upon the foundation of traditional qigong.

Concepts of Health Qigong

Qigong was first brought under government management in China in August 1996, for the purpose of guiding the healthy development of social qigong activities. The relevant government departments jointly issued the *Notice of Enhancing the Management of Social Qigong*, introducing and defining the concepts of "Social Qigong", "Health Qigong" , and "Qigong Medical Care". "Social Qigong" is "Health Qigong and Medical Qigong activities participated in by many people". Qigong exercises participated in by people for the purpose of fitness, promoting health, and rehabilitation are Health Qigong. Qigong exercises being taught or applied directly for the purpose of medical treatment are Qigong Medical Care.

In July of 2000, the State Ministry of Health enacted the *Provisional Regulations on the Management of Medical Qigong*, in which "Qigong Medical Care" was renamed "Medical Qigong" and defined as "*treating disease with the methods of qigong*".

Then in September of the same year, the General Administration of Sports of China further defined "Health Qigong" as "a traditional national sport". In the *Provisional Regulations on the Management of Health Qigong*, it stated that "*Health Qigong is a traditional national sport mainly focusing on a combination of body movement, breathing techniques, and mental regulation; it is an important element of traditional Chinese culture.*" The Administration went on to establish an administrative agency and the Chinese Health Qigong Association to promote the popularization of health qigong. Since then, health qigong has undergone a continuing process of formalization.

Key Elements of Health Qigong Practice

A human being is composed of body and mind. The harmonious coordination of the two is necessary for health as well as meeting the purposes of qigong practice. In qigong theory, our body and mind are represented by "(physical) body" and "spirit" respectively, with qi linking the two to form an organic whole. Therefore, the life of a person is a unity of body, qi, and spirit (sometimes referred to as "body, qi and mind"), as has been written: "*Body, the residence of life; qi, the supplement of life; spirit, the governor of life* (形者，生之舍也；气者，生之充也；神者，生之制也)".

Thus, health qigong incorporates three techniques of regulation; body regulation, breath regulation, and mind regulation; which correspond to the body, qi, and spirit of a human being. The "Three Regulations" are the key elements of health qigong practice.

Body Regulation

"Body regulation" is the active and conscious regulation of the body's postures and movements to achieve the purposes of qigong. It is the foundation for breath regulation and mind regulation, and the basis of health qigong practice. Techniques in traditional qigong practice, such as "train the body by *dao-yin*" and "dignify the physical appearance", belong to the category of body regulation.

▪ Methods of Body Regulation

Body regulation includes the regulation of the body trunk and the limbs, but it does not stop there. Every part of the body, including head, neck, shoulders, elbows, wrists, palms, fingers, chest, abdomen, sides, ribs, spine, back, waist, buttocks, hipbones, legs, knees, ankles, feet, toes, eyes, ears, nose, and tongue, has detailed requirements specified for its regulation. As an example, an exercise may specify "standing in silence, relaxed", "neck and spine straightened", "sink the shoulders and elbows", "waist relaxed", "sink the hips", "tongue touching the upper palate", "eyes gazing forward". All exercises, whether dynamic or static, involve the regulation of the entire body in such a manner.

▪ Requirements of Body Regulation

The basic requirements for body regulation is proper posture and relaxation of the body, whether in walking, standing, sitting (including natural sitting posture, cross-legged sitting posture, and kneeling posture), lying (including lying on the back, lying on the side, and half lying posture), or with movements of bending, stretching, bending forward, bending backward, shaking, rotating, running, and jumping. All postures and movements should be properly performed, smooth, comfortable, soft, relaxed, skillful, consistent, and attentive.

Effects of Body Regulation

- Body regulation forms the basis of breath regulation and mind regulation. There is an old saying, *"Qi cannot circulate smoothly if the shape is improper; mind will be restless if qi cannot circulate smoothly; spirit will be scattered if mind is restless* (形不正则气不顺，气不顺则意不宁，意不宁则神散乱)". This points out the role of body regulation as the basis of practice, for only when the body is relaxed and properly aligned can the qi be at peace and the spirit be contained.

- Body regulation softens the sinews and strengthens the bones, which makes the body strong. *"Movements promote the digestion of food and the circulation of blood, so that diseases will not be caused* (动摇则谷气得消，血脉流通，病不得生)".

- Proper body regulation techniques free the channels and collaterals and promote blood circulation, which links the human body into a unified whole. Only when the channels and collaterals are free and unobstructed can qi and blood circulate normally to maintain the life and health of a person.

Breath Regulation

Breath regulation involves actively and consciously regulating and controlling the breath in terms of frequency, rhythm, and depth. Breath regulation is an important element in the practice of health qigong. In traditional qigong, practices such as *tu-na* (exhalation and inhalation), *lian-qi*[11], *tiao-qi*[12], *fu-qi* (qi taking), and *shi-qi*[13] (qi eating) all belong to the category of breath regulation.

Methods of Breath Regulation

There are many ways to regulate the breath in health qigong. Here, we introduce several common techniques.

- Natural breathing: For health qigong beginners, except for specific requirements in the routines, the best choice is to use natural breathing, inhaling and exhaling through the nose. One can gradually achieve the unity of body, qi (breath) and mind by simply applying natural breathing in conjunction with consistent qigong practice.

- Nasal inhaling and mouth exhaling: This technique is usually used when it is needed to make a sound while exhaling, and in the relaxation phase before starting to practice a routine.

---

11. *lian-qi*: Qi training or qi exercising, a term that refers to qigong practices in general and sometimes refers to a specific type of qigong practice.
12. *tiao-qi*: Qi adjusting, a term that refers to qigong practices in general and sometimes refers to a specific type of qigong practice.
13. *shi-qi*: Qi eating, a traditional practice of qigong.

- Abdominal breathing: The common breathing techniques can be classified into thoracic breathing and abdominal breathing. Abdominal breathing can be further classified into cis-abdominal breathing (or simply abdominal breathing) and reverse abdominal breathing. With cis-abdominal breathing, bulge the abdomen naturally on inhaling and contract naturally on exhaling. On the inhale, the abdominal muscle relaxes, the diaphragm muscle drops, and the abdominal wall gradually bulges; on the exhale, the abdominal muscle contracts, the diaphragm muscle rises, and the abdominal wall returns to normal or becomes slightly concave. With reverse abdominal breathing, the belly contracts naturally on the inhale and bulges naturally on the exhale. On the inhale, the abdominal muscle and abdominal wall contract while the diaphragm muscle contracts and drops, reducing the abdominal volume. On the exhale, the abdominal muscle relaxes, the abdominal wall bulges, and the diaphragm muscle rises, increasing abdominal volume. Reverse abdominal breathing massages and exercises the internal organs and is especially helpful for improving gastrointestinal function.

- Breathing with anus contracted: On the inhale the sphincter and perineum muscles contract and lift, and on the exhale they drop; this is usually used together with reverse abdominal breathing.

Requirements of Breath Regulation

The basic requirements for breath regulation are that the breath be even, consistent, fine, soft, long, and deep. It is important to allow nature to take its course, proceeding step by step, avoiding mechanical copying and deliberately pursuing specific results. Breath regulation should be applied on the foundation of a properly posed and naturally relaxed body (body regulation) and a quiet and peaceful mind (mind regulation). After sufficient practice, the body, qi, and spirit will be in harmony. Once this happens, the breath will naturally achieve the desired qualities.

Effects of Breath Regulation

- Breath regulation is a critical element for both body regulation and mind regulation. On the one hand, maintaining a proper posture and a relaxed body allows one to be leisurely. On the other hand, being leisurely allows the breath to be smooth, the posture to be proper, and the body to be relaxed.

- By exhaling the used and inhaling the fresh, breath regulation refreshes the body. Breath regulation exercises promote the respiration function, allowing the body to inhale fresh qi from nature and exhale turbid qi from the body in a more effective way. Promoting the fusion of prenatal qi and postnatal qi within the body, improving the circulation of qi and blood, helps to regulate the functions of the tissues and organs, especially the respiratory system, and enhances vitality.

- Breath regulation promotes the circulation of qi and blood. Respiration is the power for the qi circulation within the body, and qi is the power of the blood circulation; it is said that "*qi is the commander of blood, blood is the mother of qi* (气为血之帅，血为气之母)." Therefore, breathing exercises promote the generation and development of qi within the body, and the circulation and distribution of blood throughout the body.

➤ Breath regulation enhances and strengthens the *zang-fu* (viscera and bowels). The saying *"exhaling with heart and lungs, inhaling with liver and kidney* (呼出心与肺，吸入肝与肾)" refers to how different methods of breathing influence the function of the corresponding *zang-fu*. Modern medical research indicates that frequent deep breathing exercises can increase the flexibility of the diaphragm muscle as well as promote the function of the internal organs, including the stomach and intestines.

Mind Regulation

Mind regulation is the active and conscious regulation of mental activities, attention, and thoughts to achieve the purposes of qigong.

In some ways, mind regulation is the most important of the "three regulations", for it is consciousness that guides practice. All movements, postures, and breathing exercises are guided by a participating consciousness. Practices in traditional qigong, such as *yi-shou*[14] (mental concentration), *cun-si* (mind induction), *guan-xiang* (visualization and contemplation), *tiao-shen*[15] (mind adjusting), and *lian-yi*[16] (consciousness training), all belong to the category of mind regulation.

Methods of Mind Regulation

The flow of mind, consciousness, and thought is active and varied. There are many emotions, or states of mind, including joy and happiness as well as anger, gloom, anxiety, sadness, and panic. Therefore the techniques of mind regulation are also varied, but they generally fall into two categories, *yi-shou* (mental concentration) and *cun-xiang* (mind induction).

➤ *Yi-shou* (mental concentration): *"One thought instead of thousands of thoughts* (以一念代万念)". "*Yi*" is mind or consciousness, "*shou*" is not distracted; "*yi-shou*" means to pay all attention to one thing and avoid being distracted. The commonly used *yi-shou* techniques are: concentrate on a certain part of the body, such as *dan-tian* (the elixir field), *ming-men* (life gate), navel, and acupoints such as KI 1 (*yǒng quán*, 涌泉) and DU 20 (*bǎi huì*, 百会), or concentrate on something outside of the body, such as the flame of a candle, a wall, a flower or an inanimate object.

➤ *Cun-xiang* (mind induction): *"One thought restricts (rules over) the other thoughts* (以念制(治)念)". Mind induction takes place in the quiet state achieved with body regulation and breath regulation, by focusing and concentrating the mind on a predetermined "target". The "target" is a conscious and ordered thought to be used to eliminate the chaotic and distracting thoughts. The commonly used

---

14. *yi-shou*: Mental concentration, a mind regulation technique of qigong, meditation and other cultivation practices.
15. *tiao-shen*: Mind adjusting, a mind regulation technique of qigong, meditation and other cultivation practices.
16. *lian-yi*: Consciousness training, a mind regulation technique of qigong, meditation and other cultivation practices.

mind induction techniques include: focus the attention on body postures and movements; focus on the breath (such as breath counting technique, breath following technique, breath listening technique and others), focus on the mind (such as no-thought technique, imagination techniques and others); focus on a specific target (such as the ocean, the moon, the sky, a cloud, words, poetry or a piece of music).

Requirements of Mind Regulation

The basic requirement for mind regulation is to "be tranquil". No matter which technique is used (mental concentration, mind induction, focusing on breathing, or others), the final target is to achieve a relatively "peaceful and tranquil" state and the harmony of mind (*shen*/spirit), qi and body, for the purpose of strengthening the body, and promoting health and rehabilitation.

Effects of Mind Regulation

➢ Mind regulation promotes physical and mental health. The states achieved during practice, such as peaceful, calm, relaxed, happy, and joyful, are helpful for regulating and promoting psychological and physiological functioning to achieve optimal health.

➢ Mind regulation develops potential and increases wisdom. The ancients stated that, "*The key to (qigong) practice is tranquility* (练功要旨唯入静)", and "*tranquility gives birth to wisdom* (静能生慧)". Scientific study has confirmed that a "tranquil" state is helpful for developing a person's potential abilities and increasing wisdom as well as improving the flexibility of the body, the keenness of the mind, the stability of the emotions, and the abilities of attention, observation, memorization, self-control, adaptation, and strength of will.

Mind regulation, breath regulation, and body regulation, corresponding to mind, qi, and body respectively, form an interrelated and indivisible unity. Body regulation is the foundation and condition for breath regulation and mind regulation; breath regulation is the link and critical element for body regulation and mind regulation; and mind regulation is the core as well as the ultimate aim of the "three regulations". Different routines place emphasis on a different part of the "three regulations", but by strictly following the keys and specifications of each routine, one will be able to achieve harmony among the "three regulations".

Chapter 3
Health Qigong Concepts

Health Qigong & Health Cultivation

Traditional Chinese Health Cultivation

Throughout the long history of China, the Chinese people have gradually come to understand the essence and patterns of human life through continually observing and summarizing nature and the processes of disease and senility. From this continuing process has developed a system of profound and unique theory and practice regarding human health, known as Traditional Chinese Health Cultivation (TCHC).

TCHC compares well with modern health cultivation methods and is a shining star of traditional Chinese culture. It is a science specializing in the prevention of human disease, in the cultivation of both body and mind, in slowing aging, and in bringing health, long life and happiness to humankind. Throughout its thousands of years of development, generations of distinguished health cultivation experts in medicine, literature, history, philosophy, and other fields have contributed to the contents and practices of TCHC.

Qigong Health Cultivation

Qigong health cultivation is a comprehensive method of health cultivation that follows the laws of nature and is guided by the theories of yin and yang and the five elements (wood, fire, earth, metal, and water). It is based on the theoretical foundation of "channels and collaterals" and "qi mechanisms". Qigong, along with diet and medicine, is one of the three basic methods of health cultivation.

There is an ancient saying, "*heaven has three treasures: the sun, moon, and stars; earth has three treasures: water, fire, and wind; humans have three treasures: essence, qi, and spirit* (mind) (天有三宝日月星，地有三宝水火风，人有三宝精气神)". There is another saying in qigong circles, "*Practice essence, qi, and mind internally; practice sinews, bones, and skin externally* (内练精气神，外练筋骨皮)". In a certain sense, the process of practicing qigong is that of continually cultivating and preserving essence, qi, and mind. These three are interrelated and mutually developed; they both sustain and restrain each other, forming an organic whole. The coordination and unification of these three is what we call health.

During the process of qigong practice, the interdependence between mind and breath and the correspondence between mind and body will gradually lead the practitioner into a state of "*body and mind unite into one, mind and qi follow each other* (形神合一、意气相随)". In such a state, the five *zhi* (five emotions or five psychological phenomena), which refers to joy, anger, rumination, sadness, and fright, become relaxed and harmonized, while the channels and collaterals are also freed of obstruction.

Dietary Health Cultivation

Dietary Health Cultivation, also called Medical Diet, is the precursor of modern diet therapy and nutrition. The application of dietary health cultivation is based on pattern differentiation, using indicated combinations of medicinals and food, preparing and cooking them with specific procedures. In dietary health cultivation, the nature of medicinals and the taste of food are combined to turn distasteful medicinals into tasty delicacies, incorporating medical therapy, health cultivation and disease prevention into the daily diet. There is perhaps no better instantiation of Hippocrates' injunction that "your food should be your medicine and your medicine should be your food". Dietary health cultivation is a perfect combination of nutrition and medical treatment. Featuring ease of preparation, reliable effects, and an absence of deleterious side effects, it has been highly praised by doctors and health cultivation experts throughout the ages.

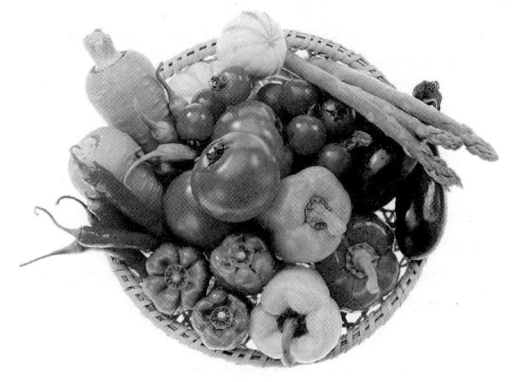

Dietary therapy can be classified in several ways. To classify by the way of cooking, there are pastries and snacks, curds and whey, pastes and drinks, steaming in clear soup, braising, steaming with ground rice, roasting, deep-frying, sautéing, stir-frying, stewing, and more. To classify by the nature of the food, there are blood and flesh, plants and trees, vegetables and fruits, mushrooms (including ganoderma lucidum) and roots, herbs and spices, and metals and stones. Dietary health cultivation emphasizes a personalized diet based on pattern differentiation; it also emphasizes the regulation of yin and yang and the five *zang* (five viscera), by using the nature and characteristics of the food and the culinary techniques to complement the needs of our body.

Medical Health Cultivation

Medical health cultivation is a key element in the overall structure of TCHC. The numerous records on the subject of the use of medicinals for prolonging life and strengthening the body go back for generations. *Shen Nong's Classic of the Materia Medica (Shén Nóng Běn Cǎo Jīng,* 神农本草经)*, Materia Medica for Dietary Therapy (Shí Liáo Běn Cǎo,* 食疗本草) and *The Grand Compendium of Materia Medica (Běn Cǎo Gāng Mù,* 本草纲目) are among the best of these works, and provide details about the variety, common knowledge, medical effects, usage, and contraindications of all types of foods and their functions in health cultivation. In *Shen Nong's Classic of the Materia Medica*, medicinals are classified into the three classes of top, middle, and low. Medicinals in the top class relax the body and prolong life, and they have anti-aging effects. Some of them boost the qi, such as *rén shēn*[17] (ginseng) and *huáng qí*[18] (milk-vetch root); some nourish the blood, such as *shú dì*[19] (prepared rehmannia root) and *dāng guī*[20] (Chinese angelica); some enrich the yin, such as *huáng jīng*[21] (sealwort) and *nǚ zhēn zǐ* [22] (privet fruit); others assist yang, such as *ròu cōng róng*[23] (desert cistanche) and *dù zhòng*[24] (eucommia bark). Since the function of the five viscera is closely related to yin, yang, qi, and blood, these medicinals have the effect of promoting and regulating the functions of the internal organs.

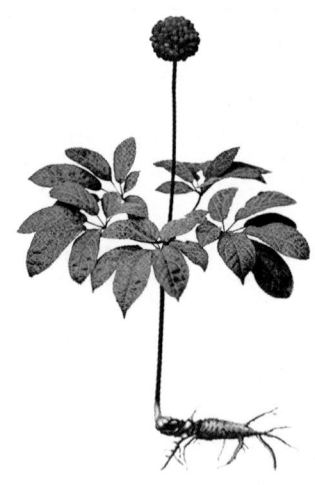

In the 21st century, people are increasingly paying attention to ways they can improve the quality and length of their lives. Chinese medicinals are becoming more and more popular, owing to their positive effects and minimal side effects. However, it is important to recognize that Chinese medicinals should not be used without the advice of appropriate counsel, which should be followed accordingly in order to prevent adverse effects caused by improper usage.

Health Cultivation according to the Four Seasons

According to the philosophy of "harmony of humans and nature", the order of people corresponds to the laws of nature. Seasonal changes, environmental changes, and other changes in nature will directly influence the physiology and pathology of the human body, especially in elders and patients suffering from chronic diseases. Such people often have reactions preceding changes in weather conditions, such as joint pain, dizziness and headache, chest distress, coughing and increased sputum, or exacerbation of their illness. Therefore, any practical health cultivation scheme must follow the

---

17. *rén shēn* (人参 , Radix et Rhizoma Ginseng, ginseng)
18. *huáng qí* (黄芪 , Radix Astragali, milk-vetch root)
19. *shú dì* (熟地 , Radix Rehmanniae Praeparata, prepared rehmannia root)
20. *dāng guī* (当归 , Radix Angelicae Sinensis, Chinese angelica)
21. *huáng jīng* (黄精 , Rhizoma Polygonati, sealwort)
22. *nǚ zhēn zǐ* (女贞子 , Fructus Ligustri Lucidi, privet fruit/glossy privet fruit/ligustrum)
23. *ròu cōng róng* (肉苁蓉 , Herba Cistanches, desert cistanche)
24. *dù zhòng* (杜仲 , Cortex Eucommiae, eucommia bark)

change of the four seasons. The changing of the seasons and weather calls for adjustments in exercise, diet, daily life, labor, and rest. Only in such a way can we achieve the harmony of yin and yang necessary for cultivating body and mind, preventing diseases, and prolonging life.

China's earliest classical medical text, *The Yellow Emperor's Inner Classic*, is highly recommended for its health cultivation advice that follows the four seasons, in which the patterns of the four seasons, the patterns of yin and yang, and the corresponding health cultivation methods are discussed. It suggests the principle of health cultivation for daily life and the mental status corresponding to each of the four seasons, which are "Birth in Spring (*chun sheng*)", "Growth in Summer (*xia zhang*)", "Harvest in Autumn (*qiu shou*)", and "Storage in Winter (*dong cang*)".

Health Cultivation in Daily Life

Good lifestyle and habits keep people healthy and long-lived, while poor lifestyle and habits do the opposite, as has been observed since ancient times.

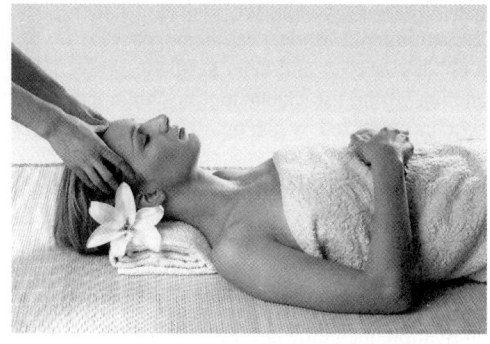

A typical person spends about one third of their lifetime sleeping. Good sleep and sleeping habits play an important role in eliminating fatigue, maintaining energy, and enhancing the body's immune system. Good sleeping conditions (e.g. bedding, room temperature and lighting) and good sleeping habits (for example, not sleeping on a full OR an empty stomach, soaking your feet in warm water before sleeping, avoiding alcohol, caffeine, and other sleep-interfering substances, choosing a comfortable sleeping position, and allowing enough time for sleeping) are highly beneficial to overall health.

A healthy diet, proper clothing, regular daily life, a comfortable living environment, and good personal hygiene are the components of health cultivation in daily life. Meeting these criteria may require us to rebuild our life patterns, develop good habits, and adjust our schedules appropriately (e.g., sleep at night, work during the day, have lunch at lunch time, etcetera).

Health Cultivation through Leisure Activities

The basic principle of health cultivation in leisure is to give your interests, hobbies, and creative activities full play. This helps to regulate your physical and mental condition and elevate mood. Choosing one or, better yet, several endeavors in alignment with your physical and economic condition can enrich life and relieve stress and fatigue.

Some of the many hobbies and interests that can be enjoyed are music, chess, calligraphy, painting, gardening, keeping pets, and fishing. From a psychological perspective, to participate in enjoyable activities adds pleasure and fullness to life.

Consider painting and calligraphy as examples. They both require a peaceful mental status, proper body posture, inspiration, creativity, comfort, and relaxation during the process. Such activities can provide mental satisfaction, assist in self-cultivation, drive off restlessness and quiet the mind, giving expression to your deepest feelings. The calligraphers in China have been known for being long-lived. On the one hand, they put their entire mind into the realm of art during the creation of a work of calligraphy. On the other hand, they must concentrate their attention on the brush and the ink, and coordinate body and mind to achieve a state of harmony through proper body posture and movement, such as suspending the elbow, lifting, pressing, and pausing. Thus, these and other so-called leisurely endeavors (such as painting and fishing) can help to develop a noble character and keen aesthetic sense, another of the life-enhancing psychological benefits conferred by qigong.

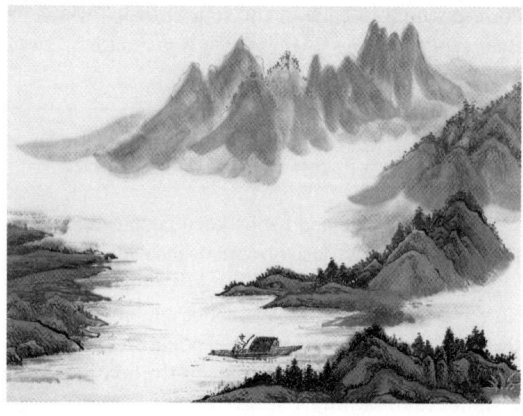

Other benefits of keeping leisure in your life include being more open-minded, optimistic, and calm. Being balanced in such a manner makes it easier to avoid emotional extremes when faced with difficulties, helping to maintain a positive mood, as well as improving overall health and slowing aging.

In addition to the above, there are also other methods and practices that can contribute to health cultivation, including martial arts and massage.

Health Qigong as the Critical Component of TCHC

There is already a large body of research on the positive health benefits of every kind of exercise. But besides the body-building functions of conventional types of sports and exercise, health qigong has several special functions. In Chapter 6 we will examine in detail the scientifically documented effects of health qigong, but here we will briefly outline the known benefits.

For Improving Physical Condition

As a traditional national sport, health qigong is not only distinct from other sports but also from other types of health exercise. Featuring soft movements and moderate exercise, it is a good sport for middle-aged and elderly people and those with weak constitutions. Besides the movements, the application of breathing techniques is another feature of health qigong, especially in health qigong *Liu Zi Jue* (The Six Sounds).

The results of preliminary scientific experiments and medical observations, as well as the feedback of long-time health qigong practitioners, have shown that health qigong has significant effects in improving the functioning of the digestive, respiratory, cardiovascular, and nervous systems, increasing appetite, releasing fatigue, improving sleep quality and blood circulation, enhancing physical strength and intelligence, and improving work efficiency and endurance.

For Disease Prevention

Health qigong boosts all of the functions of the human body. The effect of health qigong in disease prevention is achieved by strengthening the overall physique and by enhancing the body's ability to resist certain types of diseases through specific training.

Sometimes specific exercises may emphasize certain effects, such as the six sounds of "Xu", "He", "Hu", "Si", "Chui", and "Xi" in Health Qigong *Liu Zi Jue* corresponding respectively to liver, heart, spleen, lung, kidney, and *sanjiao*[25]. Health Qigong *Ba Duan Jin's* "Holding the Hands High with Palms Up to Regulate the Internal Organs", "Holding One Arm Aloft to Regulate the Functions of the Spleen and Stomach", and "Swinging the Head and Lowering the Body to Relieve Stress" are further examples. However, these effects are more generally achieved by strengthening the physique to the point where the underlying pathological condition is overcome.

Beside the effects on functional diseases, health qigong also has the effect of shortening the course of treatment of certain organic diseases (such as ulcers), by improving curative effects and promoting rehabilitation. Even more remarkably, health qigong can facilitate the effects of the treatment of many chronic and recurring diseases, freeing up people to spend more time living their lives.

For Resisting Senility and Prolonging Life

People in ancient times called qigong an art of "eliminating disease and prolonging life", saying that qigong can prevent and heal diseases as well as strengthen the body and increase the lifespan.

The results of a large number of research studies and clinical trials have shown that qigong brings people's conscious will into play in protecting themselves against disease and senility. By the practice of the "three regulations" (body, breath, and mind), the process of senility can be slowed, which is a very meaningful result for the modern studies of gerontology and geriatrics.

---

25. *Sanjiao*: One of the extraordinary *fu* organs in traditional Chinese medicine; there have been many discussions and debates over the *sanjiao* and its nature; *sanjiao* includes upper *jiao*, middle *jiao* and lower *jiao*.

For Mental Regulation and Cultivating Morals

Of the "three regulations" in health qigong, the most important and the most distinctive is mind regulation.

Health qigong adopts the principles of "*unity of mind and body* (神与形合)" and "*unity of mind and qi* (神与气合)" from traditional qigong; that is, to perfectly combine thought with movements and breathing so as to "embody mind in the body (movement)" and "embody mind in qi (breathing)". To practice with suitable music has been shown to induce happiness and relaxation. Long-term practice helps to regulate the mind and cultivate morals.

In addition, the state of tranquility in health qigong can induce the protective inhibition of the cerebral cortex, which contributes to the regulation of the internal organs and the overall function of the body, as well as enhancing the body's disease resistance. For people who stay in a peaceful and happy state, their mind and spirit are contained and not being consumed, which make them more resistant to diseases.

The goal of health qigong practitioners, then, is to strengthen the body, cultivate health, and develop a healthy lifestyle through health qigong practice.

Principles of Health Cultivation Applied in Health Qigong

Body Regulation

The principles of body regulation are "**dynamic** (movements), **tranquility** (of mind), **relaxation** (of the body and mind), and **tension** (in the application of energy and force)"; the keys of body regulation are "**proper posture**" and "**relaxation of the body**".

Cultivating Mental Tranquility: Concentrating the attention while maintaining the postures and carrying out the movements helps to achieve mental tranquility.

Regulating Yin and Yang: The dynamic gives birth to yang, while the tranquil gives birth to yin; firmness is yang, gentleness is yin. The practitioner may regulate yin and yang according to their reactions during practice, through the adjustment of the corresponding factors: relaxation and tension, firmness and gentleness, bending and stretching, or ascending and descending. All of these types of adjustments are methods of balancing yin and yang.

Regulating Qi and Blood: The "three regulations" all have the effect of freeing the body's channels and collaterals. The practices of body regulation, such as *dao-yin*, massage, and patting, have significant effects in promoting the circulation of qi and blood and strengthening the sinews and bones. This is apparent to anyone who regularly engages in qigong practice, as there is often a lingering sensation of warmth and slight sweating after practice, or even a sensation of a "warm current" passing through the body, which is what is called "the operation of internal qi (内气运行)". This effect is the natural result of developing a keen internal sensitivity. However, it shouldn't be pursued for its own sake, particularly by beginners, as this can lead the mind in the wrong direction during practice.

Softening Sinews and Strengthening Bones: With the qi and blood flowing smoothly in the body, sinews will become softer and bones will become stronger over time.

To emphasize training of the mind instead of the training of force will ultimately reduce the body's energy consumption. In one study, sixteen practitioners with hypertension who practiced qigong for over one year were monitored with ECG/EKG and medical infrared thermography. While fast-paced sports increased the heart rate of these practitioners by 35 beats per minute, some cases showed shortness of breath, chest distress, elevated blood pressure, and dimmed thermographic images of the palm. However, after practicing qigong, their heart rate increased by only 8 beats per minute, with no other uncomfortable feelings. They also showed decreased blood pressure and brightened thermographic images of the palm. These results show that health qigong not only lessens the burden on the heart but also promotes blood circulation, which makes it an excellent therapy for rehabilitation.

Health qigong practice can regulate the function of the internal organs by adjusting the relaxation and tension of the skeletal muscles, affecting the circulation and therefore the distribution of blood. Practitioners of relaxation routines and static routines tend to experience vasodilation, while practitioners of standing routines will experience vasoconstriction; practitioners of sitting routines exhibit oxygen consumption in proportion to the basal metabolic rate, while practitioners of lying routines exhibit decreased oxygen consumption, below the basal metabolic rate. Only the practitioners of standing routines have significantly increased oxygen consumption. Changes in skin temperature occur as well, most significantly with sitting practitioners, and least significantly with standing practitioners, with lying practitioners falling in the middle. One study involving five practitioners practicing static routines showed that the average basal metabolic rate decreased by 19%, with a maximum decrease of 37%. The result shows that the relaxation and tranquility engendered by qigong practice induces the inhibition of the sympathetic nervous system. Therefore, health qigong practice is effective in resisting certain harmful psychological-physiological reactions and restoring the homeostasis of the body, and thus it can effectively prevent and treat a number of psychosomatic diseases.

Breath Regulation

Calming the Mind and Cultivating Qi: Working with a foundation of natural breathing, gradually adjust the breath to make it even, consistent, fine, deep and long, which has the effect of calming the mind and cultivating qi. Abdominal breathing is frequently used for cultivating qi. It has always been believed that a large lung capacity leads to a long life.

Static routines slow the respiratory rhythm, increase the depth of breathing, and form a smooth and gentle respiratory curve, all of which contributes to improvement of respiratory efficiency. The manifestations of this improvement are increased lung capacity, increased tidal volume, and increased carbon dioxide and decreased oxygen in the alveolar gas and exhaled gas, respectively. In a study in which 21 practitioners were monitored, the average air flow of the participants' breathing decreased by 26%, while the average tidal volume increased by 78%. Likewise, the average oxygen saturation decreased from 97% to 87%, and remained in a lowered state for 10 to 20 minutes after practice was ended. These results indicate that although deep, slow respiration decreases the body's oxygen level, the coincident state of relaxation and mental tranquility lowers the metabolic rate and thus reduces the body's oxygen consumption proportionally. Simultaneously, the hematopoietic function of bone marrow is stimulated, gradually increasing the number of red blood cells, allowing the body to tolerate a lower oxygen environment.

Regulating Yin, Yang, Qi, and Blood: Inhaling corresponds to yang, while exhaling corresponds to yin. Regulating the exhalation-inhalation ratio therefore serves to regulate yin and yang within the body. For example, holding the breath and reserving the qi can serve to expel cold; exhaling the turbid qi serves to clear heat. It is found in modern medical studies that breath regulation can enhance the function of the heart, lungs, stomach, and intestines, improve the blood circulation of the internal organs, regulate the autonomic nervous system, and adjust the oxygen and carbon dioxide levels within the body, all of which are factors that improve metabolism and accumulate energy.

In the early 1980s, a newspaper in the former Sovier Union, the *"Labor"*, published an article entitled *"Deep Breathing Harms Health"*. The reason was explained as the imbalance of the blood oxygen and carbon dioxide levels caused by hyperventilation (sometimes referred as "overbreathing"). The significant decrease of the carbon dioxide level in the blood can cause or worsen spastic diseases, such as bronchial asthma, angina pectoris, angioneurotic headache, gastroenteropathy, and others. Organs such as the brain, heart, and kidney require an average of 7% carbon dioxide and only 2% of oxygen in the blood, but the air we breathe contains less than 1% carbon dioxide and approximately 20% oxygen. Therefore, many experts suggest that after inhaling we should hold the breath for as long as possible (ideally for over 1 minute); an inability to hold the breath for this long indicates a reduced adaptability. This practice is very similar to the method of breath regulation in qigong. It further shows that breath regulation helps the body to achieve equilibrium, and doesn't just exchange used air for fresh.

In modern physiology, it is indicated that the activities of the internal organs, which are not controlled by our conscious thoughts, are regulated by the autonomic nervous system. The signals of excitation of the sympathetic nervous system, such as increased blood pressure, increased respiratory rate, and enhanced metabolism, are called the syndromes of "excessive yang" in TCM. Signs of parasympathetic excitation, such as decreased blood pressure, decreased respiratory rate, increased salivary secretions, and enhanced gastrointestinal function, are called the syndromes of "excessive yin". The former is an active state of the body, which consumes energy, while the latter is a resting state of the body, which conserves energy. The excitation of the respiratory center is transmitted to the sympathetic nervous system upon inhalation, while the parasympathetic nervous system becomes excited and the sympathetic nervous system becomes inhibited in exhalation. As early as the 1950s, studies on the physiological effects of qigong indicated that breath regulation can regulate the function of the autonomic nervous system.

Mind Regulation

Regulation of the Equilibrium of Yin and Yang: Mind regulation is the core of health qigong practice, and its basic directive is to quiet the mind and achieve the state of mental tranquility. First of all, the "monarch" of the body, heart-*shen* (heart-spirit), should be protected from external distractions, allowing one to be fresh and healthy. It is said *"when the original shen (original spirit) is dominant, the conscious shen (conscious spirit) resigns* (元神主事，识神退位)"; that is, a state of mental tranquility allows the autonomous regulating systems of the body to function properly without interference. Therefore, health qigong practice has the effect of preserving and cultivating yin-essence, allowing the body to acquire the maximum amount of substance and energy from the external environment with the least amount of consumption.

Modern scientific experiments have shown that during qigong practice, skin temperature and skin potential rise and microcirculation is improved in the regions where the concentration is directed. When practitioners focus on the head, their blood pressure increases, and when they focus on the feet, their blood pressure decreases. American scholars have found that when a person trained in relaxation exercises visualizes the action of inflating a bicycle tire, an electromyograph (EMG) shows that the action potential of the biceps muscle will mimic the physical action. These results indicate that mental concentration and the state of mental tranquility can actively regulate blood distribution, mobilize body functions, and balance the body's various equilibria. This further supports the idea that the practice of mind regulation can regulate the balance of yin and yang in the body, leading to the regulation of the movement of qi and blood, and also regulating the functions of the internal organs. This, coupled with the result that mental activities can indirectly govern the activities of the internal organs through action on the autonomic nervous system, indicates that we are quite capable of self-regulating many physiological functions that are often considered to be out of our control, by reflexive attention and mental suggestion techniques such as mental concentration and mental tranquility. Generally speaking, moving thoughts are yang and still thoughts are yin; concentrating on the "outer scene" can eliminate fire, while concentrating on the "inner scene" has the effect of warming and nourishing. For example, hypertension patients should focus on KI 1 (*yǒng quán*, 涌泉), while patients with hypotension should focus on DU 20 (*bǎi huì*, 百会); people with yang deficiency should visualize "warm" scenes such as fire and the sun, while people with yin deficiency should visualize scenes with the opposite qualities.

Mental concentration practice and the achievement of mental tranquility have effects that are measurable by an EEG. The exercising EEG pattern of people who have practiced qigong for ten years or more is noticeably different from non-practitioners. In addition, the studies of experimental psychology show that the mind regulation exercises in qigong practice can improve cognitive functions such as feeling, perception, and memory. Other qualities that are measurably improved are flexibility and speed of movements; mental keenness; and the abilities of attention, observation, memorization, self-control, emotional stability, and willpower. The longer a person practices qigong, the greater the improvement in these areas becomes.

Building a Healthy Lifestyle: The aim of mind regulation is controlling behavior to develop a healthy lifestyle. As it is said, *"Tranquility is the source of wisdom* (定静生慧)", which can lead to enlightenment, allowing a person to perceive clearly both that which is within and that which is outside of the body. The consequent improvement in cognitive ability makes controlling behavior become even easier. In the terminology of health qigong, this dynamic is summarized as a balance of mind, diet, and exercise. It has long been the opinion of the ancients that people who can coordinate the balance of these elements tend to live long and healthy lives, and these same principles have been put into practice by the WHO in the form of its "Victoria Declaration", which describes the "FUN" lifestyle:

F—Frequent exercise: five minutes preparation time, twenty minutes exercise time, five minutes settling time, three to five times per week. Target: after exercise, pulse = 170/min – age.

U—Unison and harmony: a harmonious, intimate, and caring family relationship, with communication and understanding.

N—Nutrition: a simple and balanced diet with a wide variety of green food.

Chapter 4

Introduction to Health Qigong Routines

The Four Health Qigong Routines

In order to promote the popularity and ease of transmission of health qigong as a component of Chinese culture, the Chinese Health Qigong Association organized a group of experts to condense the best of the traditional qigong routines into four new standard health qigong routines. These four routines are called Health Qigong *Yi Jin Jing* (The Classic of Sinews Changing), Health Qigong *Wu Qin Xi* (The Five Animals Frolic), Health Qigong *Liu Zi Jue* (The Six Sounds), and Health Qigong *Ba Duan Jin* (The Eight Pieces of Brocade), which are shortened as "One[26], Five, Six, and Eight", or even more simply "1568". In this section we will introduce these four routines.

Health Qigong *Yi Jin Jing*

"*Yi*" means change, "*Jin*" means sinews, which includes all the different kinds of tissues of the body or the body itself, while "*Jing*" simply means classics. The *Yi Jin Jing* is thus a classical text on the way of using exercise to soften, stretch, and strengthen muscles, sinews, and bones. It is a famous routine, and there are many beautiful legends about its origin. One such legend says that it was created by the Buddhist master Bodhidharma, who was the founder of the Zen school of Buddhism. The legend says that he observed that monks had the syndromes of qi stagnation and static blood caused by long periods of sitting meditation without body movements. Therefore, he developed this exercise to promote the circulation of qi and blood, to soften the sinews, and to strengthen the bones and the entire body. Some scholars, on the other hand, hold that *Yi Jin Jing* was created by a Taoist monk, Zi Ning, in Tian Tai Mountain during the years of Tian Qi in the Ming dynasty. There have been many debates on who is the real creator of *Yi Jin Jing*. However, what is well established is that the most popular *Yi Jin Jing* routine, "12 Movements of *Yi Jin Jing*", was first found in *The Illustrated Explanation of Internal Practices* (*Nèi Gōng Tú Shuō*, 内功图说), which was recorded by Pan Wei in the eighth year of Xian Feng during the Qing dynasty.

Health Qigong *Yi Jin Jing* inherits the essence of the traditional twelve-movement routine of *Yi Jin Jing*. It is rearranged incorporating the theories of qigong, TCM, and modern physical training, combining body and mind training in a single exercise. It is scientifically rigorous as well as popular,

---

26. The word "*Yi*" in the name "*Yi Jin Jing*" has the same pronunciation as number "1" in Chinese.

and it incorporates primitive simplicity along with modern concepts and understandings. The *Yi Jin Jing* routine has twelve movements, including:

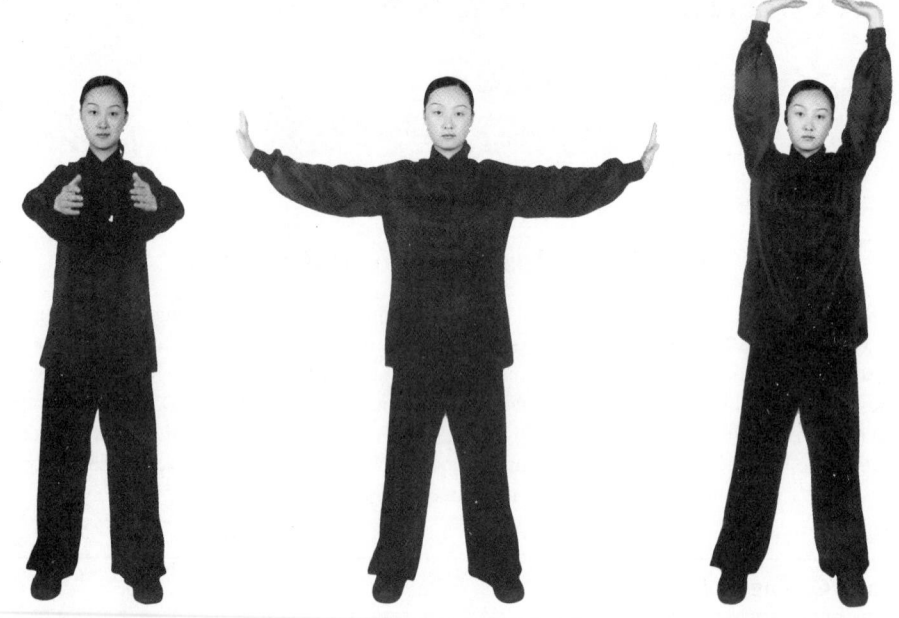

Wei Tuo Presenting the Pestle 1

Wei Tuo Presenting the Pestle 2

Wei Tuo Presenting the Pestle 3

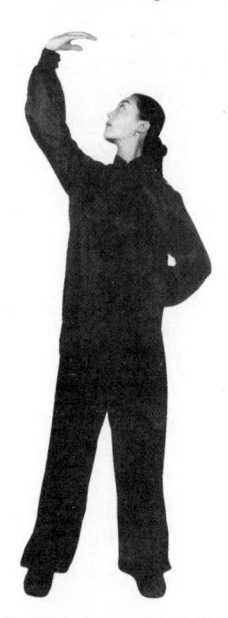

Plucking Stars on Each Side

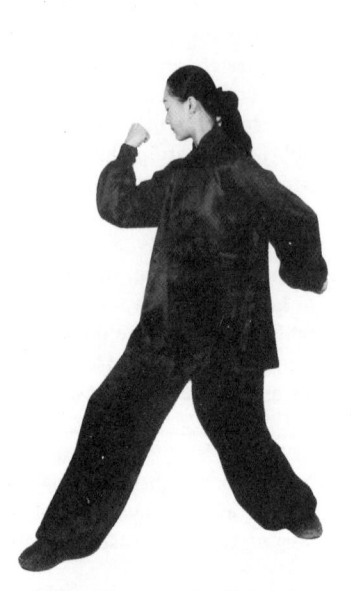

Pulling Nine Cows by Their Tails

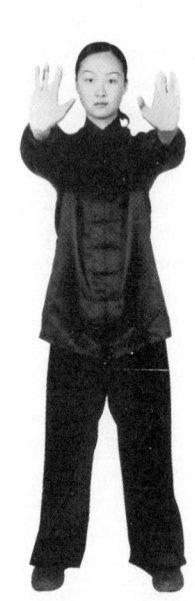

Showing Talons and Spreading Wings

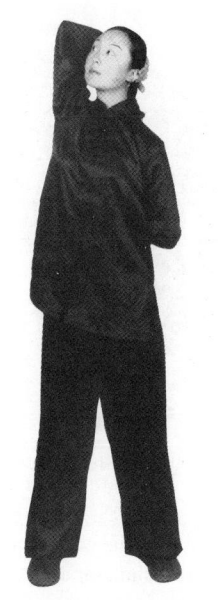

Nine Ghosts Drawing Sabers

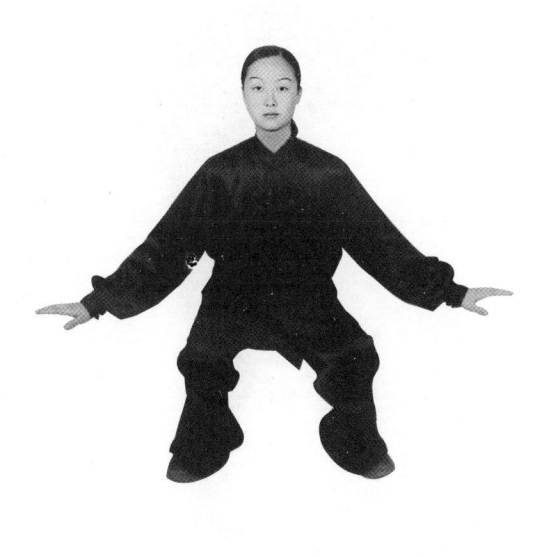

Sinking the Three Bodily Zones

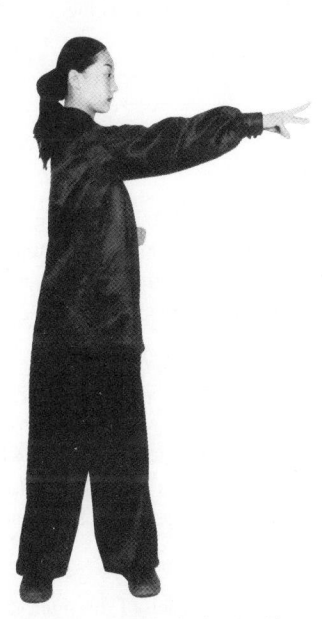

Black Dragon Displaying Its Claws

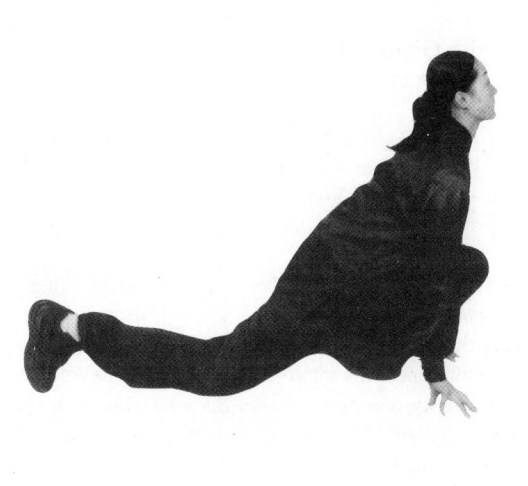

Tiger Springing on Its Prey

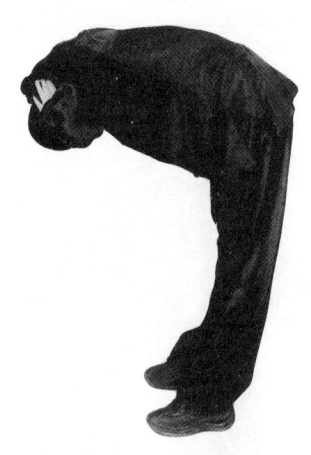

Bowing Down in SalutationSwinging the Tail

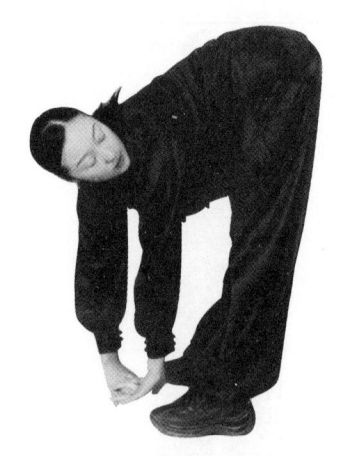

These movements are consecutive and together form an organic whole. The entire routine focuses on the rotation, stretching and bending of the spine, and also on the stretching and extending of the sinews and bones. The movements flow in a smooth and continuous way, incorporating both strength and gentleness with aesthetic appeal. Natural breathing is applied in the practice of *Yi Jin Jing*, and the breath should be in harmony with the movements. Qi and mind follow the movements of the body. Following these principles will lead to significant health benefits.

Health Qigong *Wu Qin Xi*

Wu Qin Xi (Five Animals Frolic) was created by the famous doctor, Hua Tuo, during the Eastern Han Dynasty. It was inspired by the movements of tigers, deer, bears, apes, and birds, and created on the theoretical foundations of the TCM theories of qi mechanism, channels and collaterals, and visceral manifestation, as well as the patterns of qi circulation and physiological changes.

The recording of Hua Tuo's *Wu Qin Xi* was first found in *The Chronicle of Three Kingdoms – Biography of Hua Tuo* (*Sān Guó Zhì – Huà Tuó Zhuàn*, 三国志·华佗传), written by Chen Shou during the Western Jin Dynasty. Then, the routine was described and explained in detail with both illustrations and texts in works such as *Essence of the Red Phoenix* (*Chì Fèng Suǐ*, 赤凤髓) of the Ming Dynasty, and *The Celestial Book for Long Life* (*Wàn Shòu Xiān Shū*, 万寿仙书) written by Cao Wu-ji of the Qing Dynasty. A number of schools of *Wu Qin Xi* have developed over time, each with a unique style and features.

The routine of Health Qigong *Wu Qin Xi* has five exercises, one for each of the tiger, deer, bear, ape, and bird. Each exercise consists of two movements, so there are ten movements in the routine. In addition, there is an opening movement at the beginning of the routine to settle and regulate the breath, and a closing movement at the end to lead the qi back to the origin. The routine embodies the harmony of body, qi, and mind, with the design of the movements organically combining physical aesthetics and modern kinesiology. It is based on TCM theories including *zang-fu* (viscera and bowels), channels and collaterals, and combines the characteristics of the five animals. Each of the five exercises of the routine has a specific function of its own, as well as a synergistic fitness effect. *Wu Qin Xi* displays the spirit of the five animals by imitation of their movements: the bravery and fierceness of the tiger, the quietness and elegance of the deer, the steadiness of the bear, the cleverness of the ape, and the agility of the bird. Thus, it incorporates both their shape and spirit, both mind and qi, uniting the internal and external. The movements are symmetrical, reliable and safe to practice, the routine is easy to learn, and it promotes the balanced development of health. Practitioners may practice in the range and intensity of motion which suits them individually. And, as with any other routine, the more familiar one becomes with the movements the more detailed the practice of the three regulations becomes.

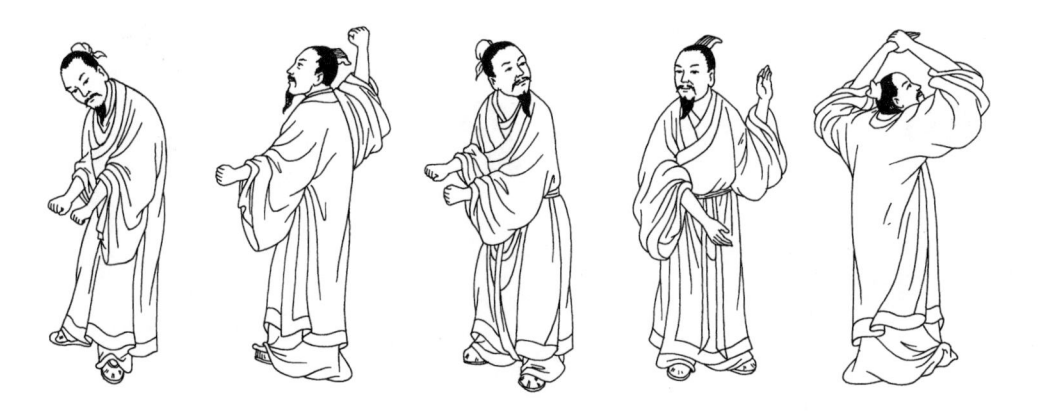

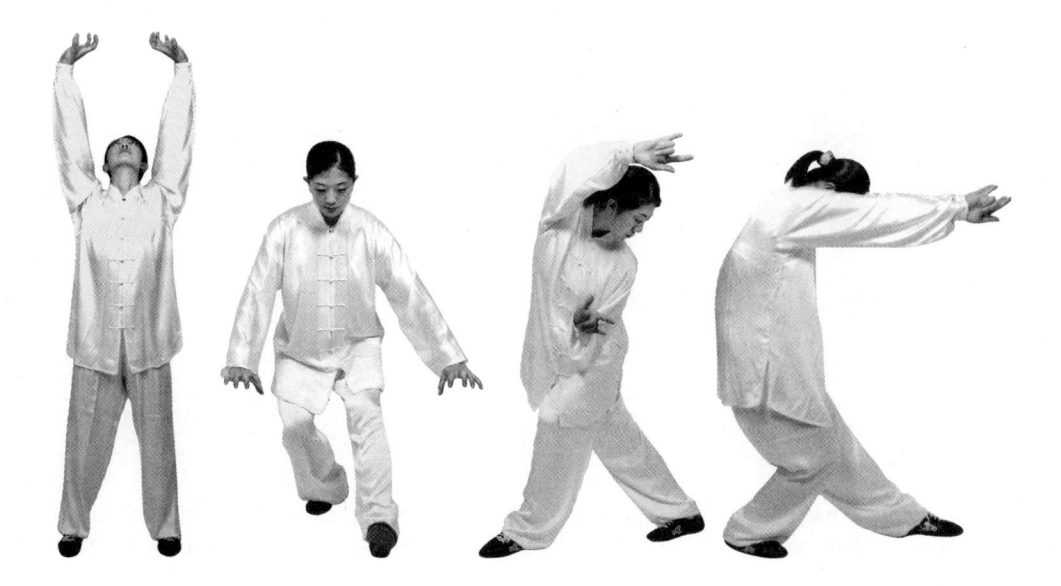

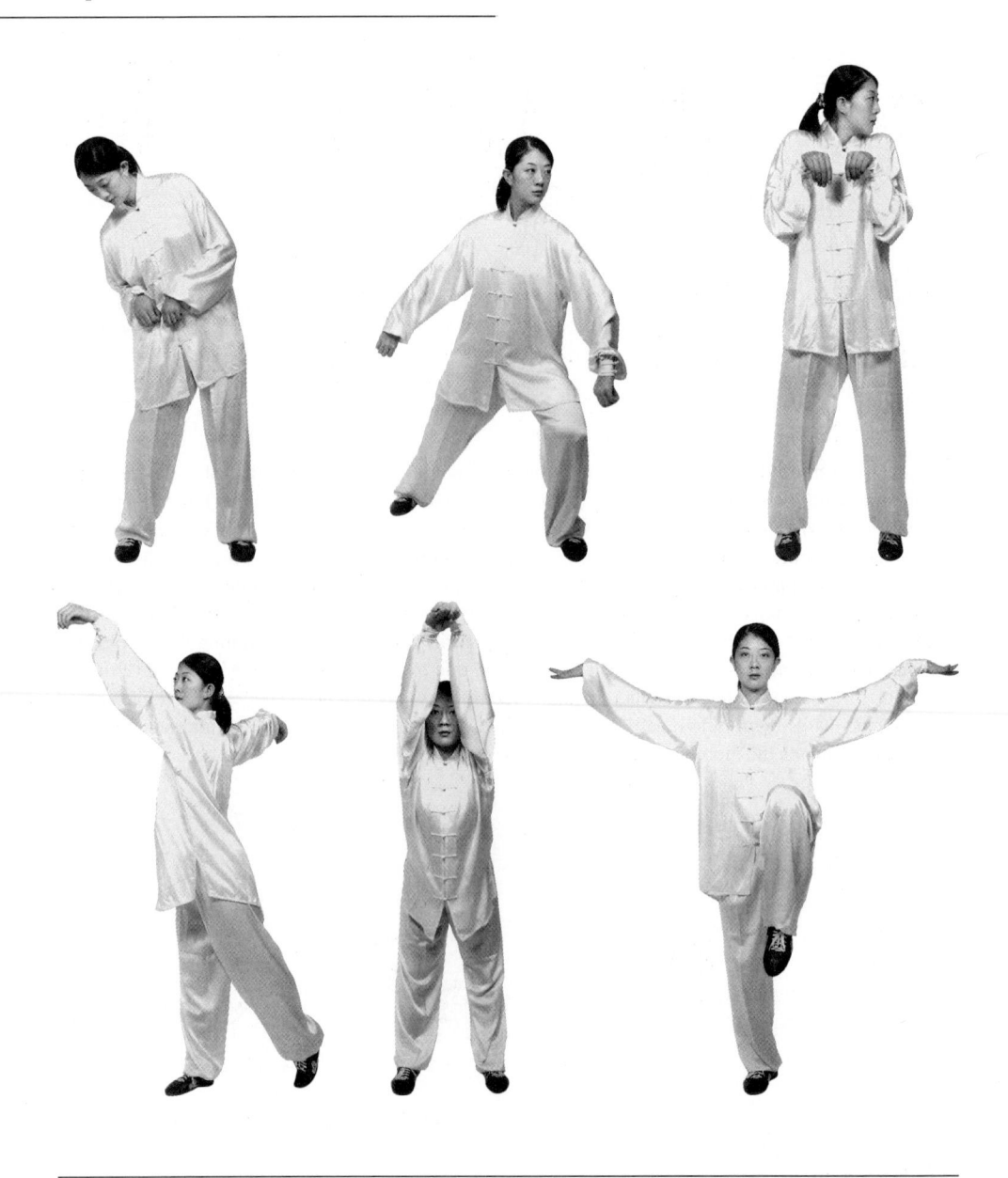

Health Qigong *Liu Zi Jue*

Liu Zi Jue (The Six Sounds), is a practice of combining the exhalation and inhalation techniques of breathing with pronouncing the six sounds of xū, hē, hū, sī, chuī, xī, in order to adjust and regulate the qi mechanisms of the liver, heart, spleen, lung, kidney, and *sanjiao*. It is a unique health exercise for strengthening the internal organs, eliminating disease, and prolonging life.

There is a long history of using pronunciation of specific sounds along with breathing techniques for the purpose of cultivating health and treating disease. It can be traced back as early as the ancient classic *Tao Te Ching/The Classic of Dao and Morals* (*Dào Dé Jīng*, 道德经). In *Records of Mind Cultivation and Life Prolonging* of the Southern and Northern Dynasties, there is a complete explanation of the six sounds: "*chuī to clear heat, hū to dispel wind, xī to relieve vexation, hē to lower the qi, xū to dissipate cold, sī to recover from fatigue* (吹以去热，呼以去风，唏以去烦，呵以下气，嘘以散寒，呬以解极)." This reflects that the six sounds had been widely used as a method of curing disease and promoting health and rehabilitation since very early in history. There are many records of *Liu Zi Jue* from the generations since, and many medical doctors and health cultivation experts have contributed to its techniques, theories, and application.

Health Qigong *Liu Zi Jue* emphasizes breathing exercises and pronunciation of the sounds, supplemented by simple body movements. The routine is simple and easy to learn, and the movements are soft and slow, incorporating both static and dynamic characteristics. It is both an internal and an external form of training. In the course of compiling the set, research was carried out and new specifications were made for the precise pronunciation of the sounds and the shape of the mouth for pronouncing each sound. The six sounds form a systematic and integrated whole, with each of the sounds independent of but supplemental to the others. Besides breath and sounds, corresponding movements are used to enhance the internal organs and strengthen the sinews and bones. The movements of *Liu Zi Jue* are comfortable, gentle, smooth and slow, like the flow of clouds and water. The routine is a combination of the dynamic and the static, having both the effect of exercise and health cultivation, with a distinctive qigong quality. There is a simple classical movement for each of the six sounds, plus the "ready position" and the "starting position" for activating the qi mechanism, and the "closing form" for leading the qi back to the origin, for a total of 9 movements. The entire routine emphasizes the principles of "qi follows body" and "mind follow qi".

Health Qigong *Ba Duan Jin*

"*Ba Duan*" has the meaning of "eight sections" or "eight pieces" in Chinese. It does not simply refer to eight sections of the routine or eight movements, but signifies that this routine is composed of many intricate elements. "*Jin*" means "brocade" in Chinese. A fine and luxurious textile woven by silk, it signifies the delicateness and preciousness of this routine. In another sense, "*Jin*" can be interpreted as a collection of techniques and instructions of *dao-yin*, which are woven together to form a comprehensive exercise, as the brocade is woven from the silk threads.

The name "*Ba Duan Jin*" first appeared in the *The Chronicle of Yi Jian*[27] (*Yí Jiān Zhì*, 夷坚志) created by Hong Mai during the Southern Song Dynasty, in the following passage: "*Year seven of Zheng-he, Li Si-ju was the imperial diarist...he woke up at midnight, did breathing exercises and self-massage,*

---

27. Yi Jian: The name of a person.

practicing what is called Ba Duan Jin (政和七年，李似矩为起居郎 …… 尝以夜半时起坐，嘘吸按摩，行所谓八段锦者)". At the end of the Qing Dynasty, in the *New Illustration of Preserving Body – The Eight Brocade* (*Xīn Chū Bǎo Shēn Tú Shuō – Bā Duàn Jǐn*, 新出保身图说·八段锦), the name of "*Ba Duan Jin*" was first used, with illustrations, to depict a complete routine of movements. While the exact origin of *Ba Duan Jin* is uncertain, it is found that there are illustrations and descriptions of similar movements and postures in both the *Daoyin Diagram* (unearthed in the Mawangdui #3 Han Tomb of Changsha, Hunan Province) and the *Records of Mind Cultivation and Life Prolonging* (written by Tao Hong-jing during the Southern and Northern dynasties), showing that there are certain connections between these works and that *Ba Duan Jin* has a rich cultural background.

Health Qigong *Ba Duan Jin* is designed in accordance with the principles of kinematics and physiology, which makes it an aerobic exercise. The movements include:

➤ Holding the Hands High with Palms Up to Regulate the Internal Organs

➤ Posing as an Archer Shooting Both Left- and Right-Handed

➤ Holding One Arm Aloft to Regulate the Functions of the Spleen and Stomach

➤ Looking Backwards to Prevent Sickness and Strain

➤ Swinging the Head and Lowering the Body to Relieve Stress

➤ Moving the Hands down the Back and Legs and Touching the Feet to Strengthen the Kidneys

➤ Thrusting the Fists and Making the Eyes Glare to Enhance Strength

➤ Raising and Lowering the Heels to Cure Diseases

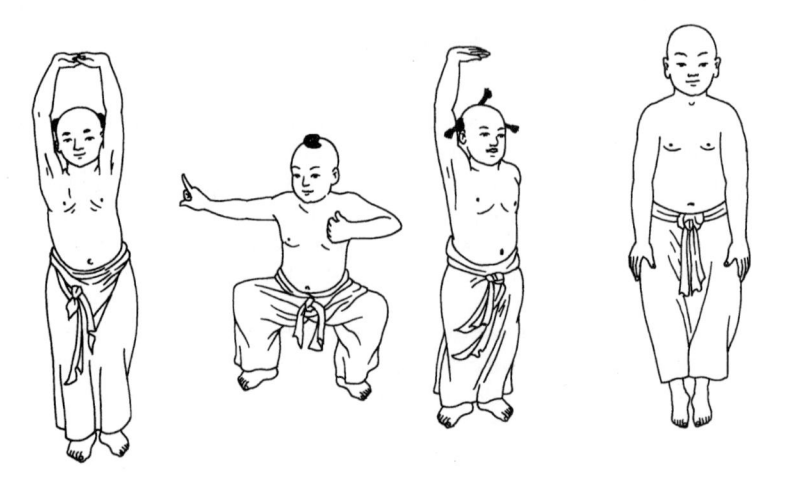

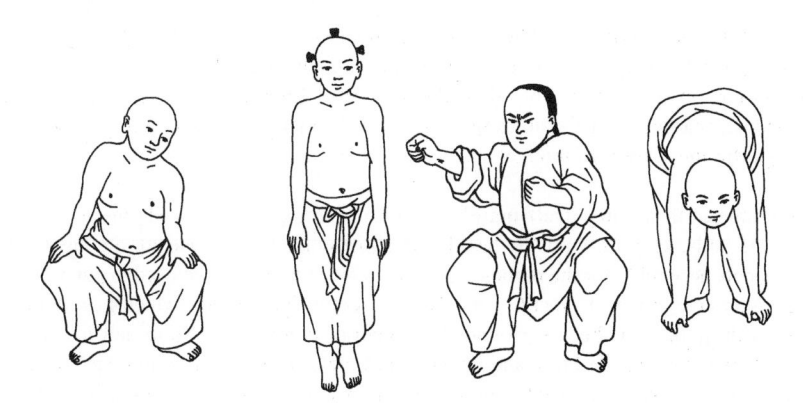

In addition to the above movements, there is a "Ready Position" at the opening of the routine and a "Closing Form" at the end, which make it a complete exercise. The entire routine is soft, slow, smooth, coherent, relaxed, natural, flexible, nimble and comfortable. It combines the characteristics of looseness and tension and the dynamic and the static. During the practice, the body should be in harmony with the mind and the qi. Each movement should be agile, coherent, and characterized by symmetry and harmony. Altogether the routine embodies the concepts of the coupling of emptiness with fullness and hardness with softness. In practice the body follows the mind, achieving the effect of overall health promotion through cultivation of the mind and training of the body.

Principles Guiding the Creation of Health Qigong Routines

The health qigong routines are the first meaningful attempt by a group of experts to create a systematic form of qigong. Their success is attributable to conceptual breakthroughs which make the health qigong routines different from traditional qigong exercises. Here we introduce some of the principles that informed the creation of health qigong.

Principles of Strengthening the Body and Cultivating Health

Among the rich cultural inheritance left by the ancient Chinese, including a long-standing history and a vast geographical expanse, is the art of qigong, which has been practiced and refined by millions of people over thousands of years, and which continues to grow in richness and diversity. Over time there have been many schools, many interests, and many value orientations applied to the development of qigong. Some have approached it from the perspective of keeping fit and promoting health, some from the perspective of curing disease, some from the perspective of self-defense and resistance against enemies, some from the perspective of improving skills and performances, and some from the perspective of pursuing immortality.

In recent decades, particularly the 1980s, the popularization of qigong led to a profusion of new qigong styles, which often led to confusion for beginners. Although all of these new styles contributed to the development of qigong, not all of them were of high quality and some were downright ignorant and superstitious. This is an example of why skepticism and scientific rigor are necessary in interpreting differing schools of thought.

The term health qigong itself mainly refers to qigong activities which can be practiced to strengthen the body, keep fit, cultivate health and assist rehabilitation. Health qigong practice should ideally be widely accessible for the purpose of promoting health, instead of used to pursue "immortality" by a small, secretive group of practitioners. The concept of immortality which has traditionally been associated with qigong has been surrounded by ignorance and superstition, not to mention elitism. Therefore, "strengthening the body and developing fitness, health cultivation, and rehabilitation" is the slogan of modern, scientific health qigong. Such a value orientation is not only practical, but also guides the development of qigong in a positive manner.

Yi Jin Jing (Classic of Sinews Changing), *Wu Qin Xi* (The Five Animals Frolic), *Liu Zi Jue* (The Six Sounds), and *Ba Duan Jin* (The Eight Brocades) are excellent representatives of the traditional qigong treasures. They emphasize either the training of body movements or breathing exercises, have significantly positive health effects, and are safe and reliable for anybody to practice, making them quite suitable for popularization.

What is more, both rigorous scientific experiments and the experiences of countless practitioners have proved the effectiveness of health qigong in strengthening the body and promoting health. The movements are easy to learn and memorize, having no complicated mental configurations or difficult, taxing movements. The duration and intensity of practice are easy to handle, especially for the middle-aged, elderly, and infirm. At the same time, the routines embody all of the challenges inherent to qigong, taking a short time to learn but a lifetime to master, allowing practitioners to progress and improve as long as they live.

Using Science as a Yardstick in the Development of Health Qigong

A wide variety of qigong styles have been around for a long time, consisting of different features and movements, but in general they all have the same aims of exercising the bones, facilitating the circulation of qi and blood, preventing and curing disease, and prolonging the life span. However, certain exaggerations, such as achieving immortality, are abundant in the literature and language of qigong. This is why the new health qigong routines were developed in accordance with scientific methodology, to allow for the accurate discernment and absorption of the relevant wisdom of traditional qigong.

Thus, the new health qigong routines were developed and studied as research topics. The chief research group responsible for the subject is the Chinese Health Qigong Association. The bulk of the research itself was awarded, after a bidding process, to Beijing Sport University, Shanghai Institute of Physical Education, Wuhan Institute of Physical Education, Xiyuan Hospital of Chinese Academy of Traditional Chinese Medicine, Beijing University of Chinese Medicine, and Capital Institute of Physical Education, resulting in the formation of four subgroups which bore the task of composing the new routines of health qigong.

The scientific method was applied to the entire process of research and development of the theories and routines of health qigong, to ensure that health qigong is a "scientific health exercise".

Chapter 5

Features of Health Qigong

Health Qigong Qualifies as Aerobic Exercise

Western philosophers have said, "sunshine, air, water, and movement are the sources of life and health." Another common saying is "Life lies in movement." However, there are many types of exercise, with a variety of intensities, effects, and forms. But which ones are the most beneficial to health? This was the question on the mind of Dr. Kenneth H. Cooper, an exercise physiologist in the United States Air Force, who together with his colleague Colonel Pauline Potts, coined the term and developed the precise method of "aerobic exercise".

"Aerobic" means "with oxygen", so aerobic exercise refers to endurance exercise that can facilitate the circulation of blood and air within the body by strengthening the heart and lungs and promoting their functions. All the tissues and organs of our body need a sufficient supply of air and nutrition to maintain an optimally functional state. The most popular types of aerobic exercises are walking, jogging, swimming, rope skipping, and biking. Although anaerobic ("without oxygen") exercise, such as static training, weightlifting, working out with certain types of fitness equipment, and sprinting, can strengthen the muscles' explosive power, they do not provide the fitness benefits of improved circulatory and respiratory function that aerobic exercises do.

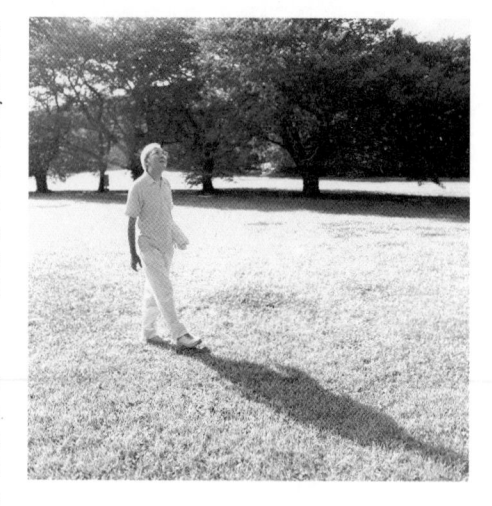

Aerobic exercise has three traits, which are intensity, duration, and frequency. The best results are achieved by exercising at an intensity great enough to sustain an elevated heart rate for a half hour or more per session, at least three times per week. The heart rate while exercising at the maximum intensity one can bear is what we call "maximum heart rate"; this is when the heart works at its maximum capacity. For people without significant disease, the "target heart rate" or "moderate heart rate" for physical exercise is when a person reach 60%–80% of the maximum, given by the formula 220 minus age, times 60% to 80%.[28] Research shows that a moderate target heart rate (i.e., 60%–80%) is both effective and safe for most people, especially those who suffer from cardiovascular disease. Needless to say, it wouldn't do for anybody, particularly those who do suffer from symptoms of

---

28. Formula of Target Heart Rate: (220 − age) x 60%~80%

cardiovascular disease, to simply blindly attempt to achieve a particular heart rate without listening to the advice of medical professionals and the signals of their own body.

The health qigong routines have the characteristics of aerobic exercise. As an example, in a study on the practitioners of Health Qigong *Wu Qin Xi* (The Five Animals Frolic), 60 people (27 male, 33 female) between the ages of 50 and 69 with no serious or chronic diseases were organized to practice *Wu Qin Xi* at least four days per week and repeat for 3–4 times each day (not less than 45 minutes). After three months of practice, the heart rates of these practitioners while practicing were monitored using heart rate telemetry equipment. The results were that males were able to achieve their target heart rate range in an average of ten and a half minutes (in a range of 3 to 13.5 minutes), with the highest heart rate of 111/min which is 14/min less than the maximum target heart rate; while females were able to achieve the target heart rate in an average of nine minutes (in a range of 3 to 12 minutes), with the highest heart rate of 109/min, which is 19/min less than the maximum target heart rate. The average time for all the practitioners together to achieve the target heart rate range was 9 minutes (in a range of 4 to 13 minutes), with the highest heart rate of 111/min, which is 17/min less than the maximum heart rate. At the end of practice, the heart rate would gradually return to normal (below the target heart rate range). Thus, for most of the duration of the exercise, the participants were at their target heart rate range, meeting the requirements of low and medium intensity aerobic exercise for people in this age range.

The research also revealed that after these practitioners had been practicing *Wu Qin Xi* for six months, the cardiac output of each pulse had increased significantly, and the rate of abnormal ECG/EKG activity during rest or after an exercise stress test had decreased significantly. Furthermore, their breathing pattern had changed noticeably, being deeper in the resting state, indicating improved gas exchange in the lungs. The results showed that the practice of Health Qigong *Wu Qin Xi* can promote the circulatory and respiratory functions, especially for the middle-aged and elderly. Further results recorded were increased warmness in the body and limbs, improved body strength and flexibility of the joints, and improved overall health status, indicating that the practitioners received all of the benefits associated with traditional aerobic exercise.

Health Qigong Emphasizes the Overall Training of Body and Mind

The goal of social development is to improve people's lives. However, in the midst of modern development lurks a serious health crisis, composed of life threatening illnesses such as AIDS and cancer on the one hand and obesity, depression, and various other mental and psychosomatic disorders resulting from a toxic and fiercely competitive social environment on the other. These illnesses of the modern world have increased significantly, mostly resulting from unhealthy lifestyles. Unknown in ancient times, they are collectively referred to as "diseases of civilization" or lifestyle diseases.

Health qigong has an important role to play in the cure and, more importantly, the prevention, of lifestyle diseases. On the basis of traditional Chinese philosophy, health qigong emphasizes the holism of humans with the environment, nature, and society, and also the holism of the individual, including thoughts and behavior. Therefore, the focus of health qigong expands beyond conventional exercise, which tends to focus merely on training the physiological functions, by emphasizing soft and slow movements coupled with regulated breathing and an attentive mind, instead of intensive and rapid exercise for a short period of time.

For example, the practice of Health Qigong *Yi Jin Jing* focuses on body regulation, guiding the movement of qi by body movements, but it implicitly requires mind regulation in order to accomplish this, while some movements explicitly call for particular types of mental regulation. For example, the third movement of the *Yi Jin Jing* routine, "Wei Tuo Presenting the Pestle 3", requires attention on the palms, while the movement "Plucking Stars on Each Side" requires attention on the "life gate" which is on the waist. Other movements specify certain imagery: in the eighth movement of "Sinking the Three Bodily Zones", imagine holding something heavy with the hands; while in the fifth movement, "Pulling Nine Cows by Their Tails", imagine gripping the tails of cows with each hand and pulling with the shoulder muscles.

Health qigong incorporates the principle of being "relaxed, tranquil, and natural" in practice. This principle applies to the mind as well as the body. Habits of thinking should be gradually adapted to be suitable to the needs of the movements, diminishing distracting thoughts, nervousness, and gloomy emotions, allowing the brain and nervous system to relax and self regulate. Such practice is helpful for getting rid of worries and releasing inner conflicts, helping us to relieve the imbalanced psychological state associated with modern society, and strengthening our minds.

In addition to individual benefits, the research in health qigong also reveals benefits that emerge when groups of people practice together, such as promoting friendship and strengthening communication. At the same time that it improves the body of the individual, it facilitates the development of relationships, helping to alleviate the loneliness and anxiety that many people experience on a daily basis.

Health Qigong is Target-Oriented, Safe and Reliable

Health qigong is a form of sport, but it is significantly different than Western sports. Although Western sports strengthen the body, they do so by aiming for goals such as "higher, faster, and stronger". Through competition they showcase the beauty and strength of the bodies of those who run faster, jump higher, and perform with better skills and more complicated movements.

Health qigong, by contrast, is a solo form of exercise that involves not only body movements but also breathing and psychological regulation. Implicitly, it does not advocate competition or pursuit of extreme limits, but rather promotes harmony among the parts of the individual and with the environment through self-exercise, with the sole intention of strengthening the body, assisting rehabilitation, and promoting health. Because of this holistic focus, by combining the physiological, psychological, and social aspects, health qigong meets the needs of medical development, sustaining both individual and social health, which has helped it to draw widespread attention and active participation.

Compared to conventional types of sports, the movements of health qigong are not difficult, the speed and rhythm are slow, and the demands on the body are light, minimizing the chances of injury during practice. And while all the health qigong routines involve all three regulations (body, breath, and mind), different routines emphasize certain areas more than others, and the whole system is scientifically designed to be maximally effective with minimal risks, rarely causing negative side effects.

According to both research results and feedback from practitioners, health qigong is safe, effective, and reliable for maintaining an optimal state of wellbeing.

Health Qigong is Easy to Practice

Each of the health qigong routines contains simple movements with easy-to-learn essentials. Each routine requires about fifteen minutes to practice and can be learned in detail from CD-ROMs and textbooks, allowing people to study on their own, and adjust the intensity and duration of practice according to their own status. The different routines of health qigong can be practiced in conjunction or individually. Certain movements in each routine can even be practiced on their own repeatedly. The practice can be done silently or with musical accompaniment. It does not need to be limited or constrained in any way, making it suitable for male and female, young and old.

Most types of conventional sports require funds to be invested in the form of equipment or gymnasium space. This can form a barrier that keeps many people from exercising. This is not so for health qigong practice however, as it can be practiced anywhere and by anybody, with no equipment necessary.

"High efficiency, fast pace" is the theme of work and life in modern society. While many conventional sports have time requirements to participate, the time requirements for practicing health qigong are very flexible. It can easily fit into and around breaks, leisure time, idle time, and first thing in the morning before getting up or last thing in the evening before going to bed. Practice is not dependent upon weather or seasonal conditions and can be determined completely by personal factors such as strength, time, and interest.

Health Qigong Inherits the Best of Tradition and Modern Times

While qigong has been a component of traditional Chinese culture for thousands of years, among the many teachings on the subject are some which are valuable for fostering health and some which preach ignorance and superstition. However, if we were to deny completely the validity of these teachings, we would be unwise. The worthwhile challenge lies in absorbing the essence and discarding the dross. This intention, along with strengthening the management of the system, are intrinsic to the purpose of health qigong.

Health Qigong Draws upon the Quintessence of Tradition

During the process of composing the health qigong routines, the subgroups researched many related documents and searched millions of words of literature to retrieve information. As examples; the *Ba Duan Jin* group collected 64 distinct editions of the *Ba Duan Jin* ranging in date from the Southern Song Dynasty to the present date; the *Liu Zi Jue* group did topical research for ancient documents in the National Library of China, the Tsinghua University Library, and the Peking University Library, and for modern documents with the help of the Periodical Database on Medical Health and Sports.

To further incorporate the essence of traditional qigong, each research subgroup held seminars on traditional qigong, discussed widely with representatives from different qigong schools, and consulted with around 200 experts who had done related studies. The research groups also went to the birthplace of each qigong routine to find clues about its origin and accurately frame its composition. For example, the *Wu Qin Xi* Group went to Bo Zhou city in An Hui province and carried out fieldwork in the hometown of its creator, the famous doctor Hua Tuo of the Eastern Han Dynasty.

On the basis of this compilation of research from literature, surveys, and experiments, as well as thorough exchanges with experts and representatives from the many different qigong schools, the research subgroups composed the basic movements of the health qigong routines and compiled a summary on the theory of each routine. The *Yi Jin Jing* routine was transmitted mostly intact, preserving the essentials of the original 12 movements and using the same names as the original. The *Wu Qin Xi* routine is composed according to the record in *The Chronicle of Three Kingdoms—Biography of Hua Tuo*, where the sequence of the movements is recorded as: tiger, deer, bear, ape, and bird. The *Wu Qin Xi* routine contains 10 movements, 2 for each animal, as recorded in *Records of Mind Cultivation and Life Prolonging* written by Tao Hong-jing; and the specifications of movements are improved upon the basis of such records as *Records of Mind Cultivation and Life Prolonging* and the *Illustrated Explanation of the Five Animals Dance* (*Wǔ Qín Wǔ Gōng Fǎ Tú Shuō*, 五禽舞功法图说).

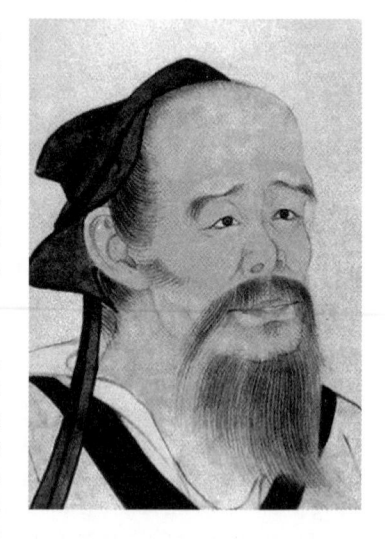

Health Qigong Meets the Needs of Modern Times

Health qigong both inherits the best of tradition and fully embodies the spirit of modern times. The theory of health qigong not only coincides with the traditional theories of qigong and TCM, but also with modern scientific methods and knowledge. It promotes traditional culture and values as well as modern scientific ways of exercising.

Although the movements of health qigong routines come from traditional qigong practices, they contain many modern components which make health qigong a special form of exercise. For example, in the *Yi Jin Jing* routine, transitional movements were added to the traditional 12 movements, thus clearing and smoothing the routine. It emphasizes how the rotation and bending of the spine drives the movement of the limbs and the internal organs as well as the coordination between the upper and lower body, between the limbs and the trunk, and between the left and right, resulting in harmonious movements that embody comfort, coherence, and beauty by artfully combining the dynamic and static phases of the human body under the guidance of a spiritual intention. Furthermore, health qigong meets the requirements of high efficiency inherent in modern lifestyles due to its being very easy to learn, safe to practice and readily adaptable to a wide range of people.

Health Qigong Incorporates Collective Wisdom to Withstand the Test of History

The composition of the health qigong routines was a systematic project. If they had been composed by only one person, or even one field of experts, they would have been too narrow in scope to meet their goals. Health qigong has been composed with input from experts not only in TCM and qigong fields but also in related subjects. In order to design a systematization of health qigong that would withstand the test of history, it was necessary to incorporate the input of diverse experts and scholars.

Some of the subjects in which experts were either consulted or included as part of the research team were martial arts, philosophy, religion, culture, art, psychology, and biochemistry. Each one joined the research team for the purposes of preserving traditional Chinese culture and contributing their specialized expertise to the development of health qigong.

The research took place in an atmosphere of open academic collaboration and innovation, and the results were successively revised through an open feedback loop between researchers, experts, and participants.

In order to further increase the quality of the finished product, a public bidding was held to assign the production of the official audio-visual and musical accompaniment and practice clothing of health qigong. The Beijing Science and Education Film Studio and China Central Television were responsible for producing instructional multimedia accompaniment, while the Central Conservatory of Music was responsible for composing the musical accompaniment, and the Academy of Arts and Design of Tsinghua University was responsible for designing the practice clothing.

Thus, we can safely say that through the mutual effort of experts and scholars from different areas, and the application of collective wisdom, health qigong contains the essence of modern qigong. It is not only recognized and appreciated by experts and scholars, but also widely popular.

Chapter 6
Physiological Effects of Health Qigong

In recent years, much research has been carried out on the physiological effects of health qigong, including measurements of both simple and comprehensive physiological indices, such as biochemical and immune indices. All of this has added up to a comprehensive picture of the physiological effects of health qigong.

Health qigong initiated the era of scientific qigong development. During the process of composing the routines, the four research subgroups each conducted a three month teaching experiment all over China. For example, the *Ba Duan Jin* group conducted the teaching experiment in the city of Harbin of Heilongjiang province. The experiment included 9 teaching and practicing sites with 200 participants aged from 45 to 70. The experimental results showed significant improvement in many of the physiological and psychological indices of the participants, which indicates that health qigong has a positive influence on human health, especially for the middle-aged and the elderly.

To provide further scientific validation of the effects of health qigong, the China State General Sports Administration conducted a research project called "*The Study of Health Effects of the Four Health Qigong Routines*" after the routines had been composed. The project was carried out by Shanghai Institute of Physical Education, Jiangxi Province Health Qigong Administration Center, Jiangxi University of Traditional Chinese Medicine, Xiyuan Hospital of China Academy of Traditional Chinese Medicine, Beijing Sports University, Anhui University of Traditional Chinese Medicine, and the Science Research Institute of the General Sports Administration. The survey part of the project covered 5,322 participants from seven cities and provinces, and the experiment part observed 1,203 participants. The experiment was carried out strictly according to scientific experimental methodology. There were experimental groups and control groups for each health qigong routine. Each sub research group conducted three tests respectively, before the practice, 3 months after the practice, and 6 months after the practice, to monitor the health of the participants. Some research subgroups conducted one more test one year after the practice. The data recorded included over 20 physiological, psychological and biochemical variables, including in some cases EEG analysis, physiological age, HRV, and others. The results of this research demonstrate scientifically the effectiveness and applicability of the health qigong routines and their suitability for popularization.

General Effects

Qigong has long been known for its effects of strengthening the body and boosting the function of all its systems through a comprehensive training of the body, qi and mind. In this section, we will look at some of the ways that these effects have been documented scientifically.

Effects on the Nervous System

Human metabolism is mainly accomplished by an integration of the neural and hormonal regulations, which serve to regulate all of the functions and activities of the body.

In health qigong practice, owing to mental regulation training of the higher nervous system activities such as consciousness and thought, the cells of the cerebral cortex are able to rest. This leads to orderly brain activities and improves the efficiency of the brain cells, which allows the optimal functioning of the brain. Another effect is that the body regulation of health qigong relaxes all the muscles and thus decreases the tension of the sympathetic nervous system, which helps to improve mood.

In one study, the EEG shows that when people are practicing qigong, their α-wave (a type of brainwave) activity increases in the frontal lobe; other studies show that there are evoked potentials of the brain stem recorded in the hypothalamus during the qigong practice state. For practitioners experiencing tranquility, there is increased activity in the frontal lobe, creating a chain reaction which causes the brain to increase the secretion of neurotransmitters such as enkephalin, which are associated with feelings of pleasure. This facilitates the functional activities of both the body and mind and enhances the body's ability to self-regulate and maintain homeostasis. Therefore, regular qigong practice can enhance the functions of the internal organs, which are controlled by the nervous system, regulate the internal environment, and promote overall healing and prevention of disease.

Effects on the Endocrine System

The functions of the nervous system and endocrine system are closely linked, to the point of being almost inseparable. The hypothalamus is the keystone linking the two: it is both a nerve center and an endocrine gland. The hypothalamus responds to brain activities and releases promoting or inhibiting hormones, which influence the hormone secretions of the pituitary gland.

In a state of mental tranquility, the brain functions in a more orderly way, and thus the hypothalamus functions to maintain homeostasis, which leads to a state of psychological and physiological equilibrium and balance of the body. The endocrine system relies on the body's fluids to transmit its chemical messengers, hormones, throughout the body. Hormones are critical substances within the body, and play significant roles in the processes of growth, puberty, maturation, and senility.

As an example of this type of effect, the rate of atherosclerosis (the thickening of arterial walls as a result of the accumulation of fatty materials) among women rises significantly after menopause, which leads to a rise in the incidence of coronary heart disease. Also, estrogen is closely related to bone metabolism, and lowered estrogen level is an important factor in the loss of bone density of women after menopause. For men, the change of sexual hormone levels also plays an important role in the senility process. Testosterone (T) is a critical sexual hormone for men. Besides its role in accessory sex organs and secondary sex characteristics, it regulates the metabolism of protein synthesis, bone growth, and calcium metabolism.

Long-term practice of health qigong incrementally promotes and enhances the endocrine system. In a study of the effects of Health Qigong *Ba Duan Jin*, it was found that after three months of practice the estradiol (E_2) levels in elderly women increased. Similarly, the testosterone (T) levels in elderly men increased after six months of practice. Likewise, six months of practicing Health Qigong *Liu Zi Jue* was enough to increase the level of estradiol and beta-endorphin (β-EP) in practitioners' bodies' as well as testosterone (T) and growth hormone (HGH). The results show that long term health qigong practice has a regulating effect on human metabolism, and may reduce the influence of aging on the levels of sexual hormones, both of which facilitate the purpose of prolonging life.

Effects on the Cardiovascular System

According to modern medical theory, the circulation of blood is mainly controlled and regulated by the nervous system. Therefore, the three regulations of health qigong practice, which can induce a person into a state of relaxation and tranquility, help to regulate the heart rate, cardiac output, and blood pressure by regulating the autonomic nervous system, particularly by reducing the tension of the sympathetic nervous system. In addition, health qigong is effective in improving the peripheral blood circulation. Therefore, health qigong is beneficial for curing and preventing diseases of the heart and blood vessels.

Effects on the Digestive System

In a state of mental tranquility, the relative excitement of the sympathetic nervous system decreases while that of the vagus nerve increases. Since the digestive system is regulated mainly by the vagus nerve, health qigong practice may promote gastric peristalsis and reduce the gastric emptying time. In addition, digestive enzyme secretions and appetite increase, both of which contribute to improving the digestive and absorptive function of the human body.

In addition to these effects, the enhanced diaphragm activities of abdominal breathing and the increased amplitude of the diaphragm movement, coupled with the increased rate of intra-abdominal pressure change and the internal massage, can effectively stimulate the blood circulation through the internal organs, helping to regulate the functioning of the stomach and intestines by the neural reflexes of the receptors of internal organs. Therefore, long-term health qigong practice provides multiple benefits to the digestive, absorptive, and excretory functions of the body.

Effects on Hematopoiesis (The Formation of Blood)

The main composition of blood is blood cells, which mainly include red blood cells, white blood cells, and platelets, each of which has a specialized physiological function. Red blood cells consist mainly of hemoglobin, which functions to transport oxygen and carbon dioxide. White blood cells are important components of the immune system that resist and destroy intruding pathogenic microorganisms by producing antibodies and phagocytes (which engulf and digest the pathogens). The functions of the platelets are to induce the clotting of blood and to accelerate the clotting time, and also to maintain the integrity of the capillary walls.

The studies of the effects of health qigong show that after three months of practicing Health Qigong *Wu Qin Xi*, the hemoglobin and red blood cells increased significantly in the male practitioners of the experimental group, indicating that the oxygen-carrying capacity of the blood was enhanced. After six months of practice, the total number of white blood cells and platelets decreased in the female practitioners, indicating improvement in the immune function and a decrease in blood viscosity.

Effects on the Immune System

The immune system is the body's defense system. Immunity is a physiological function of self-recognition and non-self exclusion. Immune function is a representative indicator of the health and physical condition of the human body. Through suitable exercises, the function of the immune system can be improved, strengthening disease resistance capacity.

The T lymphocyte is the most numerous and most important type of immune cell. The activity of T cells is frequently used to evaluate cellular immune function. The ratio of $CD4^+$ and $CD8^+$ cells in the body reflects the state of immune balance. An imbalanced ratio of these subsets will lead to immune dysfunction. Therefore, only when the $CD4^+/CD8^+$ ratio is in an appropriate range can the immune system generate appropriate immune responses to remove the foreign objects without damaging the body itself. The NK cell is an important component of the innate immunity which plays an extensive role in the body's defenses, particularly in tumor immunity.

It is found in the observations of practitioners of Health Qigong *Wu Qin Xi* that after 3 and 6 months of practicing, the $CD4^+/CD8^+$ ratio of the practitioners increased and the number of $CD8^+$ cells decreased. Three months of practicing increased the activity of NK cells of female practitioners, and 6 months of practicing increased the activity of NK cells for both male and female practitioners. These results clearly indicate a beneficial effect of long term health qigong practice for immune function.

Specific Benefits

Besides strengthening the body overall, health qigong also has specific benefits in terms of improving health and reversing or preventing disease. In this section we will review some of the specific benefits that have been scientifically recorded.

Regulating Heart Rate and Blood Pressure

The breath regulation of qigong requires deep, long breaths, and in particular the exhale is much longer than usual. This provides the effect of stimulating the excitability of the vagus nerve and slowing the heart rate. The results of the experiments on Health Qigong *Wu Qin Xi* show that after 6 months of practice, the average resting heart rate of male practitioners lowered from 79/min to 74/min while that of females lowered from 73/min to 68/min. For the Health Qigong *Liu Zi Jue* practitioners, the average resting heart rate lowered from 78/min to 74/min. The practitioners of Health Qigong *Ba Duan Jin* likewise displayed a lowered resting heart rate after 6 months of practice.

Mind regulation during health qigong practice maintains the brain in a tranquil state, minimizing interference from the internal and external environment, which results in an increased adaptability of the heart to physical activity. It also lowers the tension of the small vessels and coronary arteries and increases the elasticity of the artery walls, which leads to the effect of lowering blood pressure. Observations of practitioners of *Ba Duan Jin* and *Liu Zi Jue* revealed lowered diastolic (relaxation) and systolic (contraction) blood pressure, indicating that health qigong can be effective for improving the health of the heart and blood vessels, especially for middle-aged and elderly people.

Improving Blood Supply to the Heart

The slow, smooth, and continuous dynamic muscular movements of health qigong can increase returned blood volume to the heart as well as strengthen the myocardial contraction, and long-term practice can improve the heart's capacity to pump blood. Studies of Health Qigong *Yi Jin Jing* found that long term practice can improve the myocardial compliance and the ventricular systolic (contraction) and diastolic (relaxation) function. The exercise stress test performed after practicing Health Qigong *Wu Qin Xi* for 3 months and 6 months showed that the practitioners' heart rates decreased after finishing biking exercise. After 6 months of practicing, the practitioners of the experimental group showed significantly decreased rates of abnormal ECG/EKG in both the resting state and after exercise. This further demonstrates the beneficial effects of health qigong for the autonomic nervous system. Because of the central role that the autonomic nervous system has in the regulation of all of the body's functions, a well-functioning autonomic nervous system can improve the blood supply to the heart and enhance its functioning.

Reversing Cardio- and Cerebrovascular Disease

Health qigong qualifies as light to medium intensity aerobic exercise. It increases the lipase activities in muscles and fatty tissues and promotes the transformation of cholesterol and phospholipids to high-density lipoproteins. It is critical for the deposited cholesterol in blood vessels to transfer to the liver for degradation, effectively preventing or slowing down the development of cardio- and cerebrovascular diseases such as arteriosclerosis, high blood pressure, and others.

The experiments on health qigong show that after 6 months of Health Qigong *Ba Duan Jin* practice, the high-density lipoprotein (HDL-C) level in male practitioners significantly improved, and the triglyceride (TG), total cholesterol (TC) and index of arteriosclerosis (AS) decreased significantly as well. In women, TG and TC decreased while HDL-C increased. These results indicate that long-term regular practice of health qigong can alter the plasma lipid and lipoprotein levels, manifesting as a decrease in the concentration of TG, TC, and LDL-C and an increase in the concentration of HDL-C, which will lead to improvement of arteriosclerosis.

Females who practiced Health Qigong *Wu Qin Xi* for 6 months showed a sharp decrease in TG levels as well as improvement in the HDL/LDL ratio, indicating that health qigong has a positive effect in improving lipid metabolism disorders.

Improving Lung Capacity

The breath regulation of health qigong practice invokes a complex physiological reflex mechanism associated with respiration. On the one hand, this mechanism deepens the tranquility of the brain, while on the other hand it enhances the oxygen exchange function of the lungs. At the same time, breathing exercise massages the internal organs, improving their function, improves the circulation of blood, and helps to regulate the respiratory center and the autonomic nervous system.

In breath regulation, practitioners should breathe in a deep, long, even, gentle, and natural way. Breathing this way improves the strength of the inspiratory muscles, and to a certain extent improves the strength of the expiratory muscles and auxiliary expiratory muscles, which leads to significant improvement of the practitioner's lung capacity. At the same time, it reduces the relative proportion of respiratory dead space, and improves gas exchange efficiency between the alveolus and capillary blood, thereby bestowing overall benefits upon ventilation function, diaphragmatic motion amplitude, respiratory frequency, and gas metabolism.

Experiments show that after 6 months of practicing Health Qigong *Wu Qin Xi*, the practitioners had significantly increased lung vital capacity, increased from an average of 2.8 L to 3.08 L for men, and from 1.95 L to 2.27 L for women. The resting respiratory frequency of practitioners was lowered after 3 months of practicing, from an average of 16/min to 15/min for men, and from 17/min to 15/min for women. The lung ventilation rate was also decreased, from an average of 8.3 L/min to 6.5 L/min for men and from 6.9 L/min to 4.6 L/min for women. It was also found in the study of Health Qigong *Ba Duan Jin* that after certain periods of practice, the lung vital capacity of practitioners increased significantly, raising from an average of 3,238 ml to 3,695 ml for men after 6 months of practicing, and raising from 1,841 ml to 2,338 ml for women. All of this data confirms that health qigong practice has obvious effects on improving the body's lung ventilation and gas exchange functions.

Slowing Aging

With increasing age, many physiological functions decline, and the complicated structure and function of the human body degrades in an irreversible way. The main physiological changes that take place include: changes in body composition, decline in muscles' working ability, changes in the skeletal system, cardiac function, and nervous system function, abnormalities of blood rheology, occurrence of autoimmune diseases, reduced stress tolerance, and more. Plenty of studies indicate that moderate exercise is beneficial for delaying aging and improving physiological and psychological functions for elderly people, preventing disease and prolonging life by improving health.

After practicing Health Qigong *Wu Qin Xi* for 3 months and 6 months, the body fat percentage of female practitioners decreased, and the bone density of both male and female practitioners increased. They also showed improvements in body bending ability and in the length of time they were able to stand on one leg with eyes closed, as well as back strength. Medium to short term Health Qigong *Ba Duan Jin* practice can decrease the circumference of the waist, hips and the body trunk by reducing the fat in these parts, as well as improve reaction time, limb strength, flexibility, balance and coordination. Long term practice of Health Qigong *Liu Zi Jue* significantly improved the physical qualities of the practitioners and their exercise capacity indices in fast walking, grip strength, and side-jumping. The postmenopausal women participating in the practice showed significant decrease in the percentage and weight of body fat.

Therefore frequent health qigong practice can effectively improve bone metabolism disorders in middle-aged and older people, as well as increase the strength of both the upper and lower limbs. At the same time it can strengthen exercise capacity and the ability to maintain balance, all the while delaying and preventing the occurrence of chronic diseases and promoting health.

Under normal physiological conditions, the generation and removal of free radicals within the body is in homeostasis so they cannot cause harm. As the body ages, homeostasis will become upset, leading to an increase in free radicals in the body as the ability to remove them declines. The activity of superoxide dismutase (SOD) reflects the body's ability to remove free radicals. Aging is also closely related to the level of lipid peroxidation. Malonaldehyde (MDA) is the index for the peroxidation level of cell membrane lipids. Thus, reduced MDA level in blood serum indicates healthy cell membranes, which slows aging. Therefore, SOD and MDA are two important physiological indices for studying methods of anti aging.

The long-term middle-aged and elderly practitioners of Health Qigong *Ba Duan Jin* showed an increase in SOD levels in their peripheral blood which will lower the MDA levels in their body. Long-term practice of Health Qigong *Yi Jin Jing* has the same effect of decreasing MDA, inhibiting the peroxidation of lipids, reducing the peroxidation damages to cells and tissues and improving the activity of SOD and its function of removing free radicals. Thus, health qigong can effectively lower free radical metabolite levels and reduce the harm they cause to the body.

Chapter 7

Health Qigong and Psychological Health

As implied by the WHO's definition, "health" encompasses psychological and social dimensions as well as physiological ones. Therefore, taking up exercise for the pursuit of health should imply the pursuit of psychological and social wellbeing in addition to physical fitness. Health qigong practice improves the practitioner's psychological state as well as physical. Also, communication and cooperation within the practice group plays a positive role in improving the practitioner's interpersonal communication skills and social adaptability.

Health Qigong and Cognitive Ability

The process of how we understand the world is an important field of study in psychology. It is referred to as "cognition" in psychology to distinguish it from "knowing" as a philosophical concept. What we generally call "intelligence" is a kind of comprehensive ability of cognition, consisting of attention, observation, memory, imagination, thinking ability, and others.

Preventing Intelligence Decline

The intellectual development of a human being progresses at a non-uniform speed. In one psychological study, three kinds of intelligence test scales were use to observe and track a group of individuals. The result showed that a person's intelligence develops rapidly before the age of 13, follow by a slower development until the peak around age 25. Intelligence levels off between 26 and 35, then it begins to decline. The overall trend of human intelligence development is an ascending phase in the beginning, followed by a maintaining phase and then a declining phase. These results indicate that the decline of intelligence is a natural process that cannot be altered. In recent years, increasing studies on dementia have revealed that the age of onset is becoming younger, which is an issue that deserves attention.

Keep in mind that the rate of cognitive development is actually different for each individual. Some people display early development but also earlier decline. For example, many people develop presbyopia in their early forties, and their hearing declines as well. Conversely, some may develop at a slower speed but decline at a later age. For example, abstract thinking is the latest cognitive ability to develop, and under ordinary circumstances it does not develop quickly until middle school age. While some people's abstract thinking ability starts to decline at an early age of 50, some people are still quite active abstract thinkers in their sixties or seventies, and strongly creativity. Similarly, there are differences in the rate of development of senility between individuals. This is not merely due to congenital factors such as heredity (which do play a role), but also to behavioral factors such as learning to use the brain effectively, continually absorbing new knowledge, maintaining a sound mind, and exercising both the body and mind, all of which are factors in slowing physical and mental decline.

After 3 months of practice of health qigong, the elderly male practitioners had improved in their ability to distinguish numbers and symbols and perform mental arithmetic. After 6 months of practice, the reaction speed of their body movements improved and they showed a more significant improvement in mental arithmetic. Similar results were found for the elderly female practitioners, who showed improvement in mental arithmetic ability after 3 months of practice, and significant improvement in movement reaction speed along with the ability to memorize two digit figures after 6 months. All of these measurements are key components of traditional IQ tests. Thus, the results indicated that long-term health qigong practice can effectively slow the rate of decline of intelligence associated with senility.

Improving Attention

Attention is the factor that determines whether a person can carry on every other type of psychological activity smoothly. It is impossible to comprehend an article or solve a math problem if the attention is elsewhere. Concentration, or the focusing of the attention, is required to complete these activities. In daily life, many people do not achieve their full working or studying efficiency, not because of a lack of intelligence but because of a deficit of attention, which results in an inability to bring their full cognitive potential to bear. The main symptoms of many neurasthenia patients are lack of energy and lack of attention, which causes them to have difficulty in working and studying. These are also commonly displayed in people in a condition of sub-health.

Health qigong has beneficial effects on improving attention. The mental concentration technique of health qigong requires the practitioner to actively focus the mind on specific things or on certain parts of the body while actively excluding other types of thoughts. Such kinds of selective mental concentration are, by definition, "attention". The state of mental tranquility achieved through qigong practice is measurably different from the ordinary waking conscious state or mental resting state; it is different from both the sleeping state and the state of mental inactivity. Mental tranquility is a special psychological state, of which the features are simplified mental activity, decreased or eliminated distracting thoughts, constant concentration of the attention, a peaceful mind and emotional stability, feelings of comfort and delight, and diminished reactions to both internal and external stimulation. Thus, the improvement of the attention that accompanies health qigong practice, coupled with the corresponding improvement of physical condition and vitality, can improve the practitioner's working and studying efficiency, bestowing equal benefits to confidence and work and study habits.

Promoting Imagination

The practice of health qigong invokes the power of the imagination as well as the attention by means of training methods such as eliminating distracting thoughts, achieving mental tranquility, guiding internal qi, and actively relaxing the body, all of which require imagination. Certain exercises invoke the imagination in specific ways, such as the tiger exercise of Health Qigong *Wu Qin Xi*, which evokes the image of a majestic tiger in the remote forest preparing to hunt. Other examples are the bird exercise of *Wu Qin Xi*, which evokes the image of an extraordinary crane spreading its wings to fly by the riverside; and the monkey exercise, which evokes the image of a clever and vigorous monkey climbing and swinging freely in the forest.

Imagination is the process of refining and rearranging the images within our mind. The imagination activities in qigong practice constitute training for the brain, to activate the brain cells and thus slow the decline of brain function. The study on Health Qigong *Yi Jin Jing* found that after 6 months of practice, elderly practitioners showed a significant slow down of aging, while the control group showed normal aging speed.

Health Qigong and Mood Regulation

Everybody has emotions and desires; as long as we are alive we are full of sensations and affections. Emotions are a part of the process of experiencing the world, from happy to sad to worried to afraid. Mood is the index of a person's psychological and emotional state. Although we all want to be happy, it is inevitable for all of us to experience negative emotions such as pain, worry, fear, and sadness. The habitual experience of negative emotions has deleterious effects on health.

The Influence of Emotions on Health

An American physiologist, Erma, once designed an experiment to capture the exhaled breath of people into glass test tubes. When the breaths were condensed into water, the results were different depending on the emotional state of the person at the time the breath was captured. Breath from a peaceful state turned into clear, colorless water, while breath from the sad state had a white deposit. Even more interesting was that the breath from an angry person condensed into water with a purple deposit, which proved to be lethal when injected into a rat. Erma's explanation was that the physiological reaction to anger will activate the toxic substances within the body, which could erode the body's defense systems and immune function and cause people to become sick. This hypothesis has been supported by an investigation of employed people in Japan, which shows that those who lose their tempers often, those who are highly aggressive, and those who are depressed have lower activity of anticancer immune cells, while a positive mood is a miraculous drug to cure diseases.

The reason that emotion is so closely related to health is the physiological changes involved in the formation of emotions. In a state of extreme emotion, there is a great tension of the whole body and mind, causing negative changes from the respiratory to the circulatory to the digestive to the endocrine system, from the metabolism to the muscle tissue. These changes will induce imbalances in body functions. Concerning this issue, TCM lists seven internal causes (joy, anger, anxiety, rumination, sadness, fear, and terror) and emphasizes the close relationships between afflictions of the internal organs and abnormal emotional factors (extreme or persisting emotions).

Wishing a good mood for ourselves and others comes naturally, and we always try to avoid negative emotions. But there are always unexpected storms, and in life there are unpredictable changes. Since we cannot avoid the setbacks of life, negative moods are inevitable.

Contemporary health psychology holds that a mentally healthy person is not a person who is always in a happy mood, but a person who is optimistic in most circumstances. Just as the base line temperature of the human body is 37 degrees Celsius, but there are always minor fluctuations, the base line mood of a healthy person is optimism, and when negative moods occur the person can be expected to adjust themselves and recover quickly. This ability to regulate emotions is an essential characteristic of a mentally healthy person. Learning how to regulate emotions is an effective way to promote psychological health.

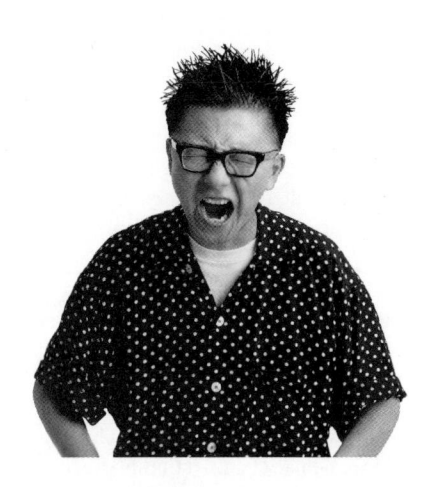

The Influence of Health Qigong Practice on Mood

Long-term health qigong practice improves the emotional stability of a person and releases mental stress and tension. One exercise that accomplishes this particularly effectively is the first movement of Health Qigong *Yi Jin Jing*, "Wei Tuo Presenting the Pestle 1". The posture of holding the palms in front of the chest can calm the emotions and contain the mind. Another example is the ninth movement in the same routine, "Black Dragon Displaying Its Claws", which helps to regulate liver function as well as ease the mood.

Studies of sports psychology found that different types of exercise can have different effects on the body. For example, bicycling, swimming, and jogging significantly improve the cognitive function, but the traditional sports of China such as qigong and *tai ji quan* are more beneficial for improving mood. After 3 or 6 months of practice, the comprehensive evaluation of the psychological state of health qigong practitioners showed different levels of improvement in mental health indicators including fear, depression, anxiety, hostility, and interpersonal relationships.

Not only does the practice of health qigong improve mood, but the learning process itself also has positive effects on the whole being.

The health qigong routines contain the essence of traditional Chinese culture. Although the movements are simple, they take time and effort to learn, particularly for beginners in middle age or older who do not know anything about qigong. Practicing the health qigong routines in an accurate and beautiful way provides a positive mental and physical challenge.

Consider the animal movements of Health Qigong *Wu Qin Xi*, which require not only regulation of the physical shape, but also understanding of the spirit and charm of the animals, in order to achieve the harmony of body, qi, and mind. It is actually quite a challenge to learn to do all of this well together. But of course, the satisfaction and pride that accompanies the accomplishment is proportional to the difficulty. This sense of satisfaction and accomplishment compounds the beneficial effects of the practice itself, bringing confidence and other positive psychological influences to the practitioners.

Psychological Explanation for Health Qigong's Effect on Mood

The "three regulations" of health qigong are consistent with the "three-factor theory of emotions" of contemporary psychology, which holds that the formation of emotion is determined by environmental events (stimulus factors), physiological state (physiological factors), and cognitive processes (cognitive factors). Among these factors the cognitive is the key which determines the nature of the emotion. For example, a person who sees a tiger (stimulus factor) will react according to various cognitive factors, such as whether the encounter takes place in a zoo or in a deep forest. Different emotional responses will then lead to different physiological responses.

Mind regulation involves regulating thought and cognition in order to achieve a state of mental tranquility. There are many different techniques of mind regulation, mostly related to the act of changing one's cognition (concepts), such as using verbal suggestions like "relax" or "quiet". This is one reason that health qigong is beneficial to psychological health.

Breath, the only physiological internal organ function that can be regulated by conscious control, can be regulated in rhythm and depth to achieve specific effects. By techniques such as body movements and mental suggestions, body regulation and breath regulation practices can relax the body and smooth the breath as well as lower the activity of the autonomic nervous system, which has the effect of regulating mood and mental state.

Health Qigong and the Optimization of Personality

Personality is the personal characteristic most closely related to society, and thus it contains social and moral elements. Personality reflects the attitude of people towards reality and the world around them and is typified by behavior. For example, when someone is in trouble, some people are inclined to offer help, while some are inclined to be indifferent, and others are inclined to seek a profit from the misfortune. Such inclinations are manifestations of a person's basic attitude, or personality.

Personality also reflects one's moral quality and is influenced by the person's views of value, life, and the world. This is why some people are selfless and some are selfish. Therefore, personality is not a constant but is gradually formed and somewhat adaptable.

Cultivation of Morals

Since ancient times qigong has been practiced not simply to strengthen the body and prolong life for its own sake, but also as a means of pursuing a noble state of refined sentiment and self cultivation. The core philosophy of health qigong is the unity of humans and nature, which implies that practitioners should consciously obey this philosophy, cultivate morals, and work to improve their character. It also follows from this that practitioners should cultivate a healthy lifestyle and seek a happy psychological state and harmonious interpersonal relationships. A stable mind under the influence of noble principles helps the practitioner to relax, release stress, and be tranquil in qigong practice; it is also the guiding principle that leads the body unerringly to a state of optimal wellbeing, and is the aim of health qigong.

Only by consciously cultivating moral values in every moment and everywhere, by applying the philosophies and principles of health qigong to daily life, is it possible to maintain a tranquil mind and a harmonious mood. Qigong cosmology, in alignment with TCM and traditional Chinese philosophies, places human beings within the cosmos and nature as well as within the social environment. It holds that we humans should follow the patterns of nature and the universe, that environmental factors, seasonal changes and social factors are connected with humans and mutually influence each other. Long-term health qigong practice therefore molds the temperament while strengthening the body.

Effects on Type A Personality

Medical and psychological studies have revealed personality to be an important basis of mental and physical health. It is also a factor in both mental and physical diseases, influencing everything from the chances of getting a particular disease to the length of its course and more. Character is an indispensable part of personality, and personality is the intermediary between stress and health, which determines whether we are carefree or whether we worry ourselves into a state of illness under the same stress. Research into the relationship between Type A personality and mental and physical health has drawn a lot of attention.

The definition of Type A personality stems from the heart disease research of two American scholars, Freidman and Rosenman, who divided human behavioral traits (personality and character) into the two categories of Type A and Type B. Type A individuals can be described as fast acting, impatient, irritable, highly competitive, ambitious, time-conscious, perfectionist, and always rushing, with a tight schedule. Often those who tend towards this type of personality are frank and unintentionally hurtful in their dealings with others. Common habits, such as making indiscreet remarks and fist-shaking, can leave an overbearing impression. Type B individuals, in contrast, are described as less competitive, passive rather than aggressive, slow-paced, relaxed, patient, easy-going, tolerant, kind, fond of entertainment, and generally lacking any sense of urgency or competition.

Type A individuals have explicit behavioral patterns, such as aggressive, uncontrollable ambitions, persistent hostility towards others, a business-like mentality, workaholic tendencies, and a strong sense of time. These patterns cause them to tend towards tense, irritable, and hasty emotional states, which has effects on physical health ranging from insomnia to migraines, digestive problems, and cardiovascular disease. The national health research institute in America has even announced that Type A personality is one of the four major risk factors for heart disease, along with high cholesterol, high blood pressure, and smoking.

Psychologists suggest that people with Type A personalities should slow their pace of life, reduce the demands they place on themselves, enjoy the fruits and joy of their successes, and give less thought to personal gain, success, fame, and wealth in order to balance their state of mind and promote good health. These recommendations are in line with the philosophy of qigong practice. Both TCM and health cultivation emphasize that "it is more important to cultivate personality than to cultivate health". The Taoist philosophers Lao Zi and Zhuang Zi both advocated the principles of conforming to natural law, being content and indifferent to worldly gain, and discarding selfish desires and worries.

Thus, consistent long-term health qigong practice can contribute to overall health by reducing the neurotic tendencies in the personality and diminishing the negative influences of a Type A personality.

Health Qigong and Interpersonal Relationships

Although there is no globally accepted standard of psychological health, there is a common understanding that it involves good interpersonal relationships.

Interpersonal Relationships and Mental and Physical Health

Interpersonal relationships play a critical role in an adult's life. Harmonious relationships with family, colleagues, friends, and neighbors are integral to a person's sense of happiness, fulfillment, and security. This idea is captured in the Chinese sayings "a fence needs the support of three stakes, and so a good man needs the support of others", and "as children we depend on our parents, and as adults we depend on our friends". A person without the support of others tends to feel lonely, helpless, and distressed, which has a diminishing effect on psychological and physical wellbeing.

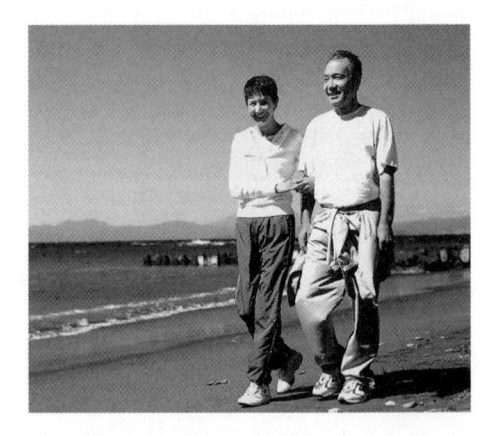

Interpersonal relationship quality is also closely related to length of lifespan. In an American study, the researchers spent 9 years tracking 6,900 adults in California, of which 8% died during the course of the study. Analysis of their data relating to social relationships revealed that those who had better interpersonal relationships had a lower mortality rate compared to those who were more isolated.

One important way that good interpersonal relationships can positively influence health is by providing proper information and emotional support for people trying to improve their health. Family and friends can help one to break bad habits and improve behavior patterns. People living in solitude are more likely to smoke or drink, for example, because they are unable to receive advice, support, and comfort from others, even if they want to make a change.

Factors Affecting Interpersonal Relationships

Many people are perplexed by the problems of how to build good interpersonal relationships, how to love and be loved, and how to accept and be accepted by others.

The situational factors influencing interpersonal relationships are appearance, capability, distance, frequency of contact, and more. Personality, however, is the strongest factor. Appearance plays an important role in the beginning of a relationship but less as communication increases, while personality increases in importance. As it is said in an old Chinese saying, "as distance tests a horse's strength, so time reveals a person's heart". Personality plays a much stronger role than anything else in creating deep and long-lasting friendships.

Health Qigong's Influence on Interpersonal Relationships

The influence of health qigong on interpersonal relationships is indirect. Only when one achieves a harmonious internal state by practicing health qigong can we see the influence on the person's interpersonal relationships.

Physiology is the material basis of mental function and behavior, and improving one's own physiological and psychological state tends to reduce interpersonal friction and thus to improve interpersonal relationships. Besides promoting health and curing and preventing disease, health qigong practice can improve the wellbeing of a person in the sub-health state and improve or even cure the symptoms of a person with physical or mental illness. These improvements will help to reverse the decline of the mental state and thus effectively improve tense interpersonal relationships. For example, inadequate sleeping patterns and insufficient energy can make people more prone to lose their tempers and be quarrelsome, which can be helped by correcting the underlying physiological imbalances.

Health qigong also improves interpersonal relationships by optimizing a person's personality through the cultivation of morality and the development of a noble mind. Noble-minded people are more patient and tolerant, tending to socialize well with others and have a kind heart, which is the most important factor in creating harmonious interpersonal relationships.

Health Qigong as a Platform for Communication

Health qigong has the further effect of bringing practitioners together in a healthy social setting. China, like most of the developed world, is becoming an aged society, particularly in certain cities like Beijing and Shanghai. The traditional multi-generational extended family households of China have been turning into small families with a few family members only, leading to the increasing number of "empty nest" households. Decreased contact with family members and others, particularly after retirement, leaves many older people feeling lonely, which has a detrimental effect upon their physical and psychological health.

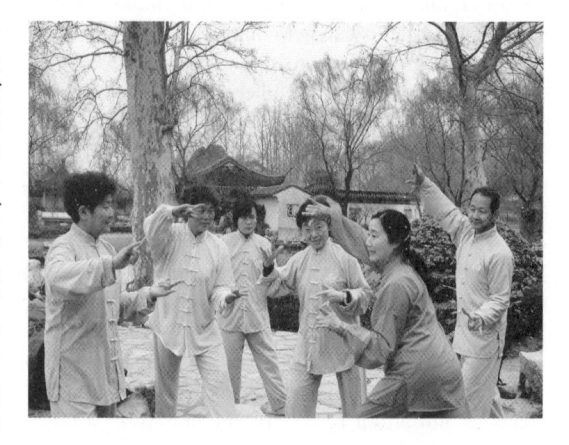

Health qigong practice not only provides a path for practitioners to manage and master their own bodies, it also provides a platform for communication, a social group, and language all of its own. As they enjoy sunshine and exercise, the practitioners also share understanding and communication about the ups and downs of life. Particularly among practice groups of similar age, there is no generation gap, and they tend to find many common topics of discussion. The friendships formed broaden communication circles and strengthen social support. The exchange of thoughts and feelings disperses loneliness, as in the saying "plant a willow unintentionally, yet it yields pleasant shade". Though it may be an unintended benefit, the relationships formed through long-term health qigong practice provide fun and companionship, which itself directly improves the quality of life.

Health Qigong and a Healthy Lifestyle

As we have mentioned, health qigong practice can improve the overall functioning of the body and of the nervous system, but beyond this, its effects diffuse to every aspect of the practitioner's daily life, influencing not only the physiological and psychological state of the practitioners but also their attitude toward others, which helps promote the harmonious development of society.

The WHO's definition of health is more than a good physical body, it also includes a peaceful state of mind and social relationships. An abundance of evidence points towards the fact that health qigong, by unifying the individual internally and externally, can help move people towards optimal health and a happy and harmonious life.

The Importance of a Healthy Lifestyle

Lifestyle refers to the ways in which people go about engaging in their activities. According to a Russian study, the quality of health depended only 15% on medical factors and 85% on lifestyle factors. The WHO classifies the proportion of different factors influencing health and lifespan as 60% lifestyle, 15% heredity, 10% social, 8% medical, and 7% climatic.

Therefore, by any measure lifestyle exerts the most important influence on health and longevity. Lifestyle makes the biggest difference between a high quality of life and health and suffering from disease and early aging.

Cardiovascular disease and cancer are the leading causes of death in the developed world. An investigation of 240,000 Beijing and Shanghai residents found an increasing incidence of high blood pressure. A study of the autopsy results of over 300 deceased persons between the ages of 15 and 39 sampled from Beijing, Nanjing, and Ningbo revealed that 75.2% of the Beijing cases had coronary sclerosis, which happens to be four times the rate of Southerners.[29] From another study in the 1950s, cardiovascular diseases and cancer constituted only 17% of the causes of death, while infectious diseases constituted more than half of the causes of death. The incidence of these non-infectious diseases has increased continually since then and has become more common among younger people, constituting up to 63.5% of the causes of death, and rising to 64.57% and 67.73% in Beijing and Xi'an city respectively in 2000. However, there are studies showing that a healthy lifestyle will reduce rates of high blood pressure by 55%, stroke by 75%, diabetes by 50%, and cancer by one third, as well as prolong the lifespan for an average of more than ten years. From these results, no greater argument can be made for the need to change irrational lifestyle habits into sound ones.

It is therefore necessary to understand what a healthy lifestyle is. In the "Victoria Declaration" put forward by the WHO, the cornerstones of public health are "improvement of dietary habits", "eradication of tobacco use", "increased physical activity" and "alleviation of deleterious psychosocial factors", which can also be used to summarize what a healthy lifestyle is.

Health Qigong's Effects on Lifestyle

The principles of TCM and health cultivation are the key linking health qigong and a healthy lifestyle. Part of this relates directly to what has already been mentioned in conjunction with a healthy lifestyle, such as the physical movements of health qigong corresponding to the requirement for a moderate amount of exercise. Part of it is also indirect, such as proper diet and eradication of tobacco and alcohol use, which shows up in TCM and TCHC as well in the requirements of health qigong practice. Another part of it is both direct and indirect, such as the mental regulation in health qigong correspond to maintaining psychological balance.

---

29. Beijing is located in a more northern part of China than Nanjing and Ningbo.

Health Qigong as Part of a Healthy Lifestyle

Health qigong is a self training exercise using the techniques of body regulation, breath regulation, and mind regulation, all of which are guided by the principle of "*running water never grows stale, a door hinge never gets worm-eaten*"[30] and "*nothing is better than practicing movements for cultivating the body*"; in other words, good health requires movement. The basic purpose of movement in health qigong is to "*guide the qi to harmonize it, and stretch the body to make it pliable*", which are achieved by moving with "*a combination of dynamic and static*" and with the key of "*proper but not excessive exercise*" and "*rest if the exercise is too much, then exercise again after getting adequate rest*". It implicitly affirms that people should not exercise beyond their body's physical capability, and take a rest if they feel tired. The standard of exercise intensity and energy expenditure is summed up by "*sweat slightly, no panting*". As we have seen, the different health qigong routines meet the requirements of aerobic exercise. However, the practice also entails the elimination of distracting thoughts, the calming of the mood, and long, deep, and smooth breathing. Thus, health qigong has both distinct differences and similarities with other popular forms of aerobic exercise (see Table 7-1).

Table 7-1 Comparison of aerobic exercise and health qigong[31]

	Method	Psychological Features	Postural Features	Movement Features	Mechanical Features	Level of Intensity	Effects
Aerobic Exercise	Physical movement	Ordinary waking state, focus on external	Casual	Linear, discontinuous movement	Larger range of motion, with a shifting body weight	55–70%	Enhances the function of heart and lungs and the capacity of metabolism.
Health Qigong	Body, qi and mind (the three oegulations)	Tranquil state of mind, concentration on internal consciousness	Body erect but comfortable, deliberate posture	Slow, smooth, even, and continuous movement	Gentle and soft movements with little shifting of body weight.	45–70%	Frees the channels and collaterals, regulates internal organs, calms the mind and promotes intelligence, improves overall wellbeing

---

30. "Running water never grows stale, a door hinge never gets worm-eaten (流水不腐，户枢不蠹)"—a traditional Chinese saying; here, it implies that constant motion prevents the inroad of pathogenic factors.
31. Source: *A Discussion on the Chinese Gentle-Slow Health Exercises* (*Lùn Zhōng Huá Huǎn Jiàn Shēn Yùn Dòng*, 论中华绵缓健身运动), written by Tian Mai-jiu, Xu Wei-jun and Hu Xiao-fei.

Health qigong practice can improve physical wellbeing, strengthen internal organs, relax the body and mind, and shed excess body fat, making it an integral part of a healthy lifestyle. Coupled with its emphasis on adequate rest and a nourishing diet, by cultivating inner and outer together it has a distinct role to play in improving mental and physical health.

Health Qigong as a Bridge to a Healthy Lifestyle

Turning a lifetime of poor health habits into good ones doesn't usually take place overnight, but is rather a process of transition for most people. Health qigong can function for these people as a guiding principle leading to a healthier lifestyle.

Health Qigong Can Help in Quitting Unhealthy Habits

Because health qigong practitioners tend to be health conscious, they tend to pay special attention to their lifestyle habits and to be more self-disciplined. It is a common thing to hear a health qigong practitioner say "I exercise every day and don't smoke." Temperance tends to come about as a natural result of long term mind regulation practice and moral cultivation and intentional adjustment of multiple aspects of daily life.

Health Qigong as a Way of Learning about Health Cultivation

The traditional Chinese health exercises have been highly influenced by Taoism, Confucianism, Buddhism, TCM, martial arts, TCHC and other aspects of traditional Chinese culture. The most important result is that the theories of these health exercises have been intimately combined with the theories of TCM and TCHC, and all the routines have been arranged according to the principles of TCM and TCHC. These health exercises mostly emphasize regulating the post-natal by concentrating the attention on the elixir field and supplementing the pre-natal by using the waist as the center of all movements. Also, many of the movements are imitations of animals known for longevity. All of these factors help to establish the concepts of health cultivation for practitioners and lead them to live a healthy and long life.

Health qigong practice is much more than a form of physical exercise; it includes knowledge of health cultivation and a variety of philosophies which are lacking in other physical exercises. Thus, learning health qigong provides a chance for the practitioners to learn more about health. There was once a Japanese scholar said that "many have died not from diseases, but from ignorance". Therefore, we need to have more of the proper knowledge to promote health and long life.

Since health qigong is designed for the express purpose of improving health, practitioners tend to not care simply about precise techniques but more generally about accumulating broad knowledge regarding health cultivation that can make their practice more effective. At the same time, acquiring more knowledge about health cultivation tends to make practitioners more enthusiastic about practicing, for they understand more about the importance of the exercise, including the principles and techniques, making the practice more effective and giving rise to a virtuous cycle of health cultivation.

Health Qigong Leads to Psychological Balance

The mind regulation of health qigong requires the concentration of the attention, a quiet mind and calm mood, and the elimination of distracting thoughts, all of which serve to negate the effects of negative stimuli, strengthening the practitioner's ability to control his or her own emotions and resulting in a state of psychological balance.

The cultural context of health qigong is composed of principles including the unity of humans and nature, the way of harmony and moderation, the balance of yin and yang, and an emphasis on molding the temperament. The philosophy also holds that excesses of the "seven emotions" (joy, anger, anxiety, rumination, sadness, fear, and terror) are detrimental to the five *zang* (the internal organs), and a peaceful mind indifferent to external interference with few desires is ideal. These principles run throughout the exercises, encouraging practitioners to feel contented and attain a state of psychological balance.

Most practitioners of health qigong tend to value the development of moral qualities of the self. They don't strive to outdo others, they avoid extremes, act out of kindness, maintain an open mind and a good mood, keep harmonious relations with others and with the society, and have big hearts. All of these traits contribute to maintaining a balanced psychological state and a joyful mood.

Health Qigong Induces a Harmonious Society

The philosophy of health qigong connects the health and survival of the individual with the health and survival of the entire physical and social universe of which the individual is a component. *The Yellow Emperor's Inner Classic* says, "*Yin, yang and the changes of nature are the beginning and the end of everything, the origin of life and death; disasters will be caused by going against such law, severe diseases will not occur by conforming to it* (阴阳四时者，万物之终始也，死生之本也，逆之则灾害生，从之则苛疾不起)". The *Zhou Yi*[32] (*Zhōu Yi*, 周易) agrees that everything in the universe should conform to the laws of nature and so should all things human. These philosophies point to the idea that we humans must develop and regulate ourselves according to the natural law in order to maintain a harmonious relationship with the universe, if we want to improve the state of our life and health.

In the philosophy of health qigong, an individual is a part of society, and thus should form a unity with it and have harmonious relationships with other people. Through practicing together

---

32. *Zhou Yi: I-Ching or The Classic of Changes* from the Zhou Dynasty

and exchanging techniques and experiences, health qigong improves the psychosocial state of the practitioners, contributing to a more harmonious relationship with society. This acts in addition to the effects of temperament-molding and moral cultivation on the practitioners themselves.

Health qigong promotes the unity of body and mind as it cultivates both. "Body" is all of the physical parts of an individual, including skin, flesh, sinews, bones, and organs, as well as the qi and blood within the body. "Spirit/Mind" is the manifestation of vitality, including cognition, thoughts, and emotions. *The Yellow Emperor's Inner Classic* indicates that "*body is what the spirit relies on, and spirit is what the body bases on* (形为神所依，神者形所根)". In other words, the body and spirit/mind form the basis for one another. For example, the physical condition of a person is different at different ages, which leads to different sleeping patterns. This is only one of the ways in which the physical state influences the mental state. Similarly, all mental activities, especially emotions, are closely related to the functioning of the digestive, respiratory, circulatory, and endocrine systems. Therefore, TCHC has always valued practices that mold both body and mind, that combine dynamic movements and static techniques, to achieve a harmonious unity of the physical and mental.

These effects of health qigong are distinct from those of conventional forms of sports. As people gradually build up harmonious relations with nature, society, and their own beings, they naturally form healthy lifestyles.

In ancient times people said that qigong practice was for pursuing "*The Way* (Tao/Dao)". To modern people, health qigong is for pursuing "*The Way of Health Cultivation*" through a healthy lifestyle.

Chapter 8

Principles of Health Qigong Practice

Correct practice of health qigong leads to a healthy physique and increased strength, and can even cure illness. In addition, it can be of benefit to anybody, whatever their current state of wellness. Correct practice, however, requires attention to many principles. This chapter will focus on these principles.

Laying a Solid Mental Foundation

A solid mental foundation is the basis of adequate health qigong practice and consists of confidence, determination, perseverance, and a contented heart. Confidence means believing that you can. Determination means deciding that you will. Perseverance means resolving to keep going, no matter what. A contented heart means being at ease and content with the practice.

Confidence

A key distinction that sets health qigong apart from other healing modalities, such as massage or magnetotherapy, is that the patients perform the therapy themselves, rather than passively accepting the benefits conferred by a therapist. Any health modality relies on the confidence of the beneficiaries, but the passive modalities are more dependent on the experience and prestige of the therapists. Through practicing health qigong, practitioners are able to act as their own healers. This has positive effects on confidence that further compound the effects of the practice. But where does this confidence come from to begin with? In order to initiate this virtuous cycle of health, the practitioner must have some foundation of confidence to grow from. Though the practitioner may have doubts at first, as long as there is a seed of confidence to grow from, doubts will vanish as confidence increases with practice and with increasing knowledge and understanding of health qigong.

Determination

Some beginners in health qigong have only brief enthusiasm, just dabbling out of curiosity, with little determination. They may slack off in their practice if they do not detect obvious benefits fast enough, and as a result they will miss out on the benefits of consistent long-term practice. They may even quit the experience, with unpleasant memories of sore muscles in their waist and legs leaving a bad impression. People who begin in a relatively healthy state may be more prone to this pattern than people who begin in a weakened state, because they may not see progress as quickly and may be more prone to overstretch their body's limits. The functions of health qigong are achieved by gradually shaping physiological patterns, not by making drastic changes. Therefore, without a foundation of determination, a beginning practitioner may not have the opportunity to form a long-term habit of consistent practice.

Perseverance

As the Chinese saying goes, *"The Way is easy to reach but hard to put into practice and harder still to hold on to* (得道容易练道难，练道容易守道难)." There are many good qigong routines and it is easy enough to learn one of them, but persisting with the practice is a higher level of difficulty; hence the necessity of perseverance as a component of the mental foundation required to achieve the benefits of health qigong.

The power of health qigong is that it relies on the practitioner's own initiative to regulate his or her physical and mental state. It is a self-training regimen that gradually strengthens the various physiological functions of the body by specific step by step practice routines, but the effects don't manifest overnight.

Achieving ideal results requires consistent, long-term practice, and there are no shortcuts to this end. Those who begin practice in response to a state of illness may cease practicing once they feel themselves to be recovered, or a person may stop after a long period of time simply out of laziness and loss of ambition. There is an old Chinese saying that says, *"Learning is like sailing against a current, either forge ahead or be driven back* (学如逆水行舟，不进则退)." The effects that are gained by consistent practice will degrade without it. Maintaining consistent practice for six months or a year is relatively easy compared to maintaining consistent practice over a decade or over a lifetime. Yet, only such perseverance can unlock the full benefits of health qigong.

Contented Heart

Ancient wisdom and modern science both agree that health qigong can shorten the course of diseases, boost the curative effects of other treatments, and improve physical strength. It can help the ill become well and the weak become stronger.

However, it would be a mistake to think that health qigong is mysterious or miraculously able to cure all disease. To achieve the beneficial effects of practice, it must be approached with the attitude of a contented heart. The effect of health qigong on the body's healing mechanism involves a process, perhaps a long process. Being too eager to achieve results violates the principles of health qigong practice and can hinder the effects of practice. You need to be content and at ease even if you are seeking significant benefits.

In the course of practice, certain sensations may arise, such as heat, cold, numbness, twitching, distending or disturbing feelings, or a keen sensation of the circulation of the blood and qi within the body, all of which are normal sensations that can result from practice. They do not deserve undue attention or intent. Through the course of practice, practitioners with illness may also experience sensations at the location of disease or injury, such as pain or distension, which are perfectly normal phenomena that deserve no special attention and certainly do not need to be sought out. Such phenomena are a manifestation of the body's healthy qi countering the pathogenic factors. As the saying goes, "*Ignore the uncommon goings-on, and they will defeat themselves* (见怪不怪，其怪自败)." As practitioners shed their physical and psychological burdens and continue practicing, negative manifestations will work themselves out.

Principles of Health Qigong Practice

The process of learning health qigong is a process of moving the body towards a state of optimization and increased order. The speed of this process depends not only on the quality of practice but also on the quality of understanding of the principles. Here, we look at these principles in detail.

Unification of Body, Mind, and Qi

The purpose of taking up exercise is to fully mobilize the body. As a type of exercise, health qigong is no exception. It differs from conventional forms of exercise, however, in that it explicitly seeks to unify body, mind, and qi. All of health qigong practice centers around this principle.

Relaxation and Tranquility

Relaxation refers to a state of the body, which should be relaxed and free from tension during practice. Tranquility refers to a state of the mind, which should be quiet and peaceful.

"Naturalness" runs throughout the practice of health qigong: body posture and movement, breathing, mental state, mood, and manner should all be natural and comfortable. Following the guidance of "natural relaxation" and "tranquility" is an essential measure to prevent the practitioner from progressing in the wrong direction.

▇ The Significance of Mental and Physical Relaxation

Mental and physical relaxation are essential conditions for the achievement of the beneficial effects of health qigong practice, as well as for avoiding the detrimental effects of stress upon the body.

Physical relaxation is keeping the entire body (including skin, muscles, joints, organs, brain and all the other body parts and components) in a tension-free state during both stable postures and movements. On the one hand, relaxation benefits the circulation of qi and blood and reduces the burdens and energy consumption of the body, lowering the basal metabolic rate. On the other hand, it reduces the excitability of the body, diminishing interference in the cerebral cortex, which has the effect of inducing the mind into the state of tranquility, accelerating the body's processes of self-regulation.

Relaxation is good for the physique as well as for psychological and mental wellbeing. If a person often shows a benevolent, kind, joyful, easy, and smiling facial expression it mirrors a kind, generous, and peaceful inner world. On the other hand, perpetually holding a tense face in a hostile, hateful, angry or nervous configuration reflects a twisted mind, leading to the deterioration of the physical state. This is an example of the principle of the mutual responsiveness between body and mind. Relaxation in health qigong creates a foundation of positive mutual influence between body and mind.

Tranquility is Achieved through Relaxation

Becoming free from desires is a prerequisite for achieving tranquility. It may actually have been easier for the ancients to achieve a state of tranquility, with a life pattern of rising and sleeping with the sun, little travel, and few and simple interpersonal relationships and aspirations. With all of the stimulation modern people have from new happenings, new information, and an abundance of relationships and material temptations, attaining a state of tranquility may not be so easy. Fierce competition and the fast pace of change compound the difficulties.

This is the reason for the principle "*the first and most important technique of mind regulation is naturalness* (调心之法，首重自然)". This means to be joyful, peaceful, and contented in daily affairs, gradually eliminating the interfering factors and cultivating a generous and open mind. Being natural allows for relaxation, which is the way to tranquility.

Relaxation in Daily Life

Relaxation and tranquility are closely related. Mental tranquility requires complete physical relaxation, while on the other hand, tranquility can bring relaxation to both body and mind.

Relaxation should take place not only during health qigong practice but throughout daily life as well. Though the state of health qigong practice cannot be maintained constantly, we can constantly strive to be as relaxed as possible, which over time will become habitual, helping to preserve a peaceful, calm state.

Using Body Movements to Relax

When mental focus alone isn't enough to achieve relaxation, using body movements can help. As an example, try "*lying like a bow* (卧如弓)": while lying on one side, bend your upper torso slightly in the shape of a bow. This is a comfortable and relaxed posture for the human body, consistent with the principles of biomechanics. However, it requires certain techniques to relax all of the muscles, sinews and bones in such a posture, and the relaxed feeling is unlikely to be discovered by many people without proper training.

Using Language to Relax

Thinking too much can get in the way of practice, especially if you think of things that disturb you, such as frustrations at work, annoyances in life, or interpersonal disputes. Since such distracting thoughts hinder relaxation and tranquility, it is good to control them using the technique of *"one thought instead of thousands of thoughts"*, that is, focusing the concentration on just one thought to get rid of all other thoughts.

An example of this is the silent chanting method, which can be used when posing yourself in the ready posture. You might focus on silently repeating the words "quiet, quiet, quiet, ..." or "relax, relax, relax, ...", experiencing the words with your entire body, and relaxing all your body parts little by little. Skilled use of this method can make it very easy to enter a state of tranquility.

Motion (Dynamic) and Stillness (Static)

The "combination of motion and stillness" refers to the organic unity of the two opposites. In the context of health qigong, "motion" refers to the "dynamic exercises" and "stillness" refers to the "still exercises". As features of health qigong practice these are opposite of each other, yet unified.

Still exercises are those such as *tu-na* (exhalation and inhalation), *xing-qi* (qi leading), sitting meditation (usually with cross-legged sitting postures), zen meditation, elixir practices, and sitting in silence. However, the stillness in still exercises is not absolutely still, but used to emphasize the training of mind and qi. While the outside is still, the inside is dynamic; qi and blood continue to circulate in an orderly pattern inside the body under mental guidance, while the physical body appears quiet and motionless. This is the source of the saying *"practice vital essence, qi, and mind internally, practice sinews, bones, and skin externally* (內练精气神，外练筋骨皮)".

Dynamic exercises are exercises involving body movements, yet they require a calm interior to achieve tranquility. Since there are many ways for the human body to move, there are many kinds of dynamic exercises.

The combination of motion and stillness emphasized in health qigong practice corresponds to the unity of mind and body in the law of life. In a sense, a human being is a trinity of body, qi, and mind, each carrying out a specific role in the process of life. The key to health cultivation consists of *"cultivating the mind, harmonizing the qi, adjusting the shape, in order to follow the Way* (将养其神，和弱其气，平夷其形，而与道浮沉俯仰)". Dynamic and still exercises focus on and emphasize different aspects of practice, but a combination of the two is what optimizes life's overall functioning. Each practitioner should constantly adjust the balance of still and dynamic exercises according to his or her own needs and stage of progress. A proper combination of exercises will be based both on the guidance of a tutor, and the internal guidance of one's own experience.

Obeying the Laws of Nature

As integrated components of the vast tapestry of nature, humans are better off when their actions accord with natural law than when they don't. However, "obeying the laws of nature" can have many different interpretations.

The Interpretation of Nature (Naturalness)

"Nature/Naturalness"[33] refers to a critical principle that runs consistently throughout health qigong practice, and is also an important factor influencing it. It not only emphasizes pattern—the pattern of everything within the universe—but also emphasizes operation—the methods to reach the way of nature.

Thinkers since ancient times have elaborated on the subject of the law of nature. In the classic of Taoist wisdom, *Lao Zi/Teachings of Master Lao* (*Lǎo Zǐ*, 老子) it is held that *"humans follow the law of Earth, while Earth follows the law of Heaven, Heaven follows the laws of the Way, while law of the Way follows the law of Nature* (人法地，地法天，天法道，道法自然)". This means that the Way (*Tao*) is the origin of everything, and thus everything, including humans, should follow the rule of *"let things take their course, and take no action to interrupt* (自然无为)". It does not mean that there is another entity called "nature" transcendent of "the Way". There's another sentence from the book that holds, *"The grandeur of Tao, the preciousness of virtue, is not conferred but innate* (道之尊，德之贵，夫莫之命而常自然)". This also means that everything in the universe comes about naturally and spontaneously. The reason why "*Tao*/the Way" has been honored and why "*De*/virtue" has been treasured, is that "*Tao*" and "*De*" sustain all and interfere with none.

Thus, it can be seen that *"naturalness is the core* (自然为本)" is not only an expression of the fundamental position of natural law in the universe, but also indicates the principles of self-cultivation practice.

Obeying the Laws of Nature in Health Qigong Practice

During health qigong practice, as well as in daily life, all the postures and movements should be natural, whether walking, running, sitting, lying, or any other. Being natural is to be relaxed and comfortable without any pretending. Natural movements are smooth and gentle. Natural breathing is smooth, even, gentle, soft, and deep, without any oppression. A natural mental state is an easy state of mind with indistinct consciousness.

The understanding and application of the laws of nature is one of the most important factors for achieving the full benefits of health qigong practice.

---

33. Nature & naturalness (and also natural) are the same word in Chinese.

Obeying the Laws of Nature in Health Cultivation

Health qigong emphasizes the harmony and unity between humans and nature. Practitioners should actively exercise in a way in accord with the laws of nature, such as the periodic changes of yin and yang and the cycles of the four seasons, in order to maintain mental and ecological balance.

Obeying the Laws of Nature to Preserve Vitality

There are two aspects of "obeying the laws of nature to preserve vitality". One is to follow the changes in nature, such as seasonal changes, to cultivate health. The other is to cultivate health following the principles of being natural.

It is important to establish proper ideas about what it means to obey the laws of nature. The human body has both passive and active adaptations. Consider the responses to an environmental temperature change. Passive adaptations would include changing clothing to accommodate; active adaptations would include adapting to the change in temperature by improving the body's regulatory mechanisms. The two approaches are totally different and lead to different life statuses.

Health qigong advocates that people adapt actively to the changes in nature to achieve the optimization of body and vital activities. Both passive and active adaptations conserve vitality, but use different methods and have different effects. Active adaptation drives gradual advancement of adaptive capacity in an evolutionary process.

Relaxation as a Principle of Nature

Relaxation is a fundamental principle of nature. In the context of health qigong practice its purpose is to diminish nervous tension and allow for the coordination of the body's systems, facilitating a positive mental and physical state conducive to the unification of body, mind, and qi. Therefore, health qigong practice should be a process of continual mental and physical relaxation and involve smooth, natural breathing. It should not be pursued under pressure, as the nervousness produced will hinder progress. Other principles of health qigong practice include combining relaxation and tranquility, combining practice and cultivation, and proceeding gradually with unremitting effort. These principles have independent requirements, but all are necessary to ensure the best effects of practice. Only when these principles complement one another throughout the course of practice is progress maximal.

Combining Health Qigong and Health Cultivation

Health qigong practice exerts an obvious positive influence on the state of one's health, but practicing health qigong without paying attention to the principles of health cultivation in other areas of one's life is counterproductive. Health qigong should be practiced in combination with an overall health cultivation lifestyle plan in order to receive the maximum benefits from both.

About Health Cultivation

Many methods of health cultivation have been summarized by the ancients, with a wide range of effects. Health cultivation (养生) is also referred to as "preserving health", which means to maintain and protect health for the purpose of prolonging life.

Health cultivation has been widely thought and written about since the times of Lao Zi and Zhuang Zi. Ge Hong of the Jin Dynasty (265-420) put forward the health cultivation principle of "*the core of health cultivation is do not impair the body* (养生以不伤为本)".

It is believed that moderation and equilibrium are critical for everything in the universe. Extremes will result in reversion, as it said "extremes meet". The same is true for health cultivation, such as appropriate mental activities, diet, physical exercises, and sex life. These are seemingly simple issues but indeed difficult to achieve.

➢ The phrase "appropriate mental activities" refers to the normal fluctuations of emotions such as joy, anger, worry, thinking, grief, fear and others. Emotions that appear suddenly or violently or reach extremes of duration or intensity cause damage to the body and can trigger diseases or even death.

➢ The phrase "appropriate diet" means to maintain a healthy and fully balanced diet. An excessive or poorly balanced diet will cause harm to the body, so an appropriate diet includes a moderate amount and proper combinations of different kinds and different flavors (sweet, sour, bitter, pungent, salty) of foods. Certain individuals have addictions to certain types of foods or to certain flavors, and foods that are either too hot or too cold can have detrimental effects. Alcohol should also be avoided.

➢ The phrase "appropriate physical labor and sex life" means not too much or too little. Excess or deficiency, indulgence or suppression, both do harm to health. *The Yellow Emperor's Internal Classic* says "*labor the body but do not wear it* (形劳而不倦)", "*have regular living habits* (起居有常)", and "*do not work to extremes* (不妄作劳)", because "*long time looking harms the blood, long time lying harms the qi, long time sitting harms the flesh, long time standing harms the bones, and long time walking harms the sinews* (久视伤血，久卧伤气，久坐伤肉，久立伤骨，久行伤筋)". Much has likewise been written over the ages on the appropriate sex life.

Overindulgence results in a loss of vitality, which opens the door to serious illness, while total abstinence results in an imbalance of the body's yin and yang, which also affects health.

Succinctly put, any excess or deficiency can cause disease. This is why health cultivation stresses moderation and regulation in all things. "*Anything used excessively causes harm* (凡物之用极皆自伤也)", and any internal or external factor that acts out suddenly, violently, or continuously, exceeding the normal physiological mechanisms of the body, is a detriment to the body and can result in pathological phenomena.

Health qigong practice is targeted at improving the health of the human body, but cannot be fully effective unless combined with sound health cultivation practices in daily life and liberal application of self-care.

Health Qigong and a Healthy Lifestyle

Receiving the beneficial effects of health qigong requires "hard practice". However, the fast rhythm and high demands that modern life places on many people can make it a challenge to devote long stretches of time to anything, let alone exercising. Even retirees have households and families to look after.

One way to meet the requirement of "hard practice" is to mandate a certain period of time regularly for "compulsory exercise". By establishing a minimum baseline practice time you can be sure to gradually condition your body. But for those who are unable to reserve the time, this approach may not suffice.

Health qigong practice does not have to be fit into official sessions, it can take place at any time and place in daily life, and the effects are cumulative. In this way the practice can be merged organically even into the busiest of schedules.

For example, while waiting for a bus is a good time to practice the "Ready Posture", and while doing housework is a good time to practice the rotation of the tailbone from "Swinging the Head and Lowering the Body to Relieve Stress". One can also practice "Bear Exercise-Swaying like a Bear" while walking, or practice stretching the shoulders and expanding the chest from "Showing Talons and Spreading Wings" and shrugging shoulders from "Monkey Exercise-Lifting the Monkey's Paws" after sitting in front of a computer for a time. One can even practice shrinking the abdomen and contracting the anus while in the restroom.

As many practitioners have experienced, the movements of health qigong practice can and should be merged into daily life. By forming deeply ingrained habits of proper breath and body regulation, the effects of practice will accumulate gradually, day by day.

As a part of society, a person has a need to deal with all kinds of public and private affairs on a daily basis. It is our nature to label such affairs as good or bad, satisfactory or unsatisfactory, and our emotions change correspondingly. If we frequently overreact, our mental and physical health will suffer. From the perspective of TCM, any excessive or lingering emotional reaction will upset the balance of blood and qi, resulting in interruptions of the body's qi mechanism and a variety of diseases.

This is why health qigong places such great importance on moral cultivation as a component of mental regulation. Moral cultivation demands that we continuously monitor our state of consciousness in daily life, staying as close as possible to a state of quiet and indifference.

Lifestyle choices determine health. The full benefits of health qigong cannot be realized unless regular practice is complemented by a healthy lifestyle.

A healthy lifestyle includes adopting clothing to suit the seasons and climate. For example, in winter dress warmly rather than try to resist the cold.

During health qigong practice, wear loose clothing and soft shoes without heels. Maintain a balanced diet and do not overeat or undereat. Avoid unhealthy foods as well as smoking, drinking alcohol, and other unhealthful addictions. Keep indoor air fresh and not too dry or moist, and get adequate rest after physical or mental exertion.

Chapter 9

Precepts of Health Qigong Practice

Instructors and environment can provide the stimulus, but the crystallizing factors that determine how much benefit is received from practice are the practitioner's own beliefs and attitudes. There are a number of key precepts that, if internalized in the form of attitudes and beliefs, will maximize the benefits received from health qigong practice.

Discard Mental Burdens

Psychological preparation must precede practice in order to free the practitioner of mental burdens. When beginning practice there should be no pressing worries on the mind. This ideal might not be reachable right away, but can be reached through moral cultivation.

Relax Body and Mind Completely

Body and mind mirror one another, but to induce relaxation it is easier to start by relaxing the body. The reason is that a relaxed body creates the conditions for a peaceful mental attitude. Put another way, the mind cannot relax unless the body does first.

Proceed Gradually

Although the movements of health qigong are simple, mastering them takes time, and realizing the ideal state takes even more. Being overeager for results is a hindrance. Time is a key ingredient. This is the meaning of proceeding gradually.

Each of the three regulations should progress gradually. When learning the movements, advancement should happen little by little. Plenty of time should be allowed for internalizing the detailed points relating to each movement.

Breath regulation begins after the movements are memorized. Breathing and movement are brought in sync with each other in a gentle and natural way. The breath should be even, gentle, soft, long, and fluid. Achieving such a state takes continual practice over time. Being harsh with yourself or seeking daily improvements will only hinder your progress.

Mind regulation follows after breath regulation. Intentions are brought in sync with breath and movement. Thought can be heavier in the beginning, and become lighter when you are getting used to the practice. Practice eventually achieves thoughts so light they can barely be felt (commonly known as "no-thought"). Practice progresses this way, in the direction of increased synchronization of movement, breath, and thought and from heavier thoughts to lighter thoughts to no-thought.

Beginners, especially those practicing with the intention of overcoming a specific health challenge, often watch day by day and session by session for improvement to occur, but if their impatience disturbs their mental tranquility it will have a detrimental effect on progress. Therefore, it is best to practice without thinking of progress, benefits, or effects. This, ironically, is the way to progress the fastest.

Therefore, if progress is being tracked in some way it is better to do it at longer intervals of time, rather than session by session or day by day. This way the process is not rushed.

Intensity and duration of practice should be increased gradually, according to the individual's physical condition. Practicing beyond the limit of physical strength is detrimental.

The purpose of intentionally progressing gradually is to counteract overeagerness. Wanting instant success will only slow things down. Gradual advancement and perseverance complement one another.

Inject Perseverance throughout Practice

One of the most important factors for making progress is perseverance. Yet lack of perseverance is an issue difficult to overcome. Without unremitting effort progress will not be made and benefits previously gained will be lost.

Practitioners can adjust their own practice regimen under the guidance of instructors. Instructors can help teach practitioners to eliminate distracting thoughts, and practitioners can arrange place and time settings for practice that minimize their own sources of distraction.

The function of an instructor is insignificant if a practitioner cannot persist. Persistence is from the heart and cannot be pretended. Practitioners who deviate from the principle of perseverance find themselves stuck.

The principle of perseverance can be taken to heart by adopting a suitably compelling purpose for practice, one that the practitioner will not be tempted to abandon.

During qigong practice, the practitioner enters a state of consciousness that is distinct from both sleep and ordinary waking awareness, characterized by inhibition of the cerebral cortex, a special state that is distinct from both ordinary wakefulness and sleep, yet smooth and orderly. The more time one spends in such a state the more the mind and body will thrive together. However, such a condition can only be obtained gradually, through long-term practice.

Therefore, rather than setting up a particular health goal ahead of time, it is better to commit to persevere with practice and simply observe the effects over time. Establish perseverance first as the primary principle guiding your practice, and remember that perseverance cannot be established without a duration, and you will find the quality of your health increasing.

Injecting the principle of perseverance throughout your practice will strengthen your willpower, which itself is a compounded benefit of practice. In addition, being noble-minded and strong-willed makes anything easier to learn. Thus, strategically applied perseverance accelerates the body's progress in strengthening itself.

Be Intentional about Choosing Exercises

There is a wide variety of qigong exercises, and practitioners should choose from among them according to their individual needs. Though the exercises are individually easy to learn, beginners may still be at a loss when it comes to the selection of appropriate exercises.

Every health qigong exercise has advantages and limitations. They all coincide on the level of basic principles, but each exercise has a different emphasis. For example, Health Qigong *Wu Qin Xi* emphasizes imitating the movement characteristics of five animals, while Health Qigong *Liu Zi Jue* emphasizes the breath exercises.

Despite the difference in emphasis, all of the exercises have the same aim and the same means, namely to strengthen the body by regulating mind and promoting qi and blood. Yet some skills are more complicated and take more time to learn, while some are simpler and faster to learn. In addition, some are more or less suitable for different constitutions, states of illness, interests, and other conditional factors. Choosing the appropriate exercises in accordance with these factors will maximize the results of practice while minimizing the effort expended, while choosing exercises aimlessly will increase effort and diminish results, and might even have detrimental effects. For example, those who are very sick and weak should start with lying exercises before progressing to sitting or standing, as they consume less strength and are most conducive to relaxation. People of good health and constitution, however, are better off starting with standing or walking exercises.

Subdivide the "Three Regulations"

As the arrangements of health qigong are various, so are the ways of practicing. However, the "three regulations" are a common theme of all health qigong exercises. The goal of the three regulations is the unity of mind, qi, and body.

Adopting the simultaneous regulation of mind, breath and body is no mean feat to master, and beginners often experience the difficulty of attending to one regulation only to lose track of the other two. Subdividing the three regulations means practicing body regulation first by means of attention to posture, combining breath regulation when you get used to the postures and movements, and combining mind regulation when you can handle movement and breath together skillfully, to finally achieve the desired unity of spirit, qi, and body.

Each regulation can be further subdivided into smaller steps according to the state of progress of the practitioner. For example, the first step of body regulation is to learn and memorize the movements, the second step is to correct them, and the third step is to link them to the breath.

Breath regulation can likewise be broken down further. Deep and slow breathing should not be overemphasized by beginners, and can lead to dizziness, shortness of breath, and breathing difficulties if overdone. Therefore, breath should be natural at the beginning and abdominal breathing should not be applied in a forceful way. The attention should first be concentrated on the movements, then gently expanded to incorporate the mind with the movements. Further progress is driven by ideas and imagination rather than physical strength. The ultimate result of this progress will be a state of tranquility, in which body and spirit unite as though barely united, concentrate as though barely concentrated, exist as though barely existing.

Subdividing the three regulations makes complicated movements easier, reduces the difficulty of practice, and speeds up the learning process. However, in actual fact the three regulations develop mutually, simultaneously, and inalienably. Subdividing the three does not mean to separate them from one another, but to emphasize them differently in different stages of practice. Therefore, it is important to learn health qigong by following the principles, because trying to progress too quickly through the three regulations can be counterproductive. "You can't help a shoot grow by pulling it upwards", only with deep roots can leaves flourish. Only consistent, gradual progress will produce the expected effects. This way seems slow, but in fact it is fast compared to the alternative, and will over time lead to the state of "*regulate with no regulation* (无意之调)".

Stress the Features of Each Routine

Each health qigong routine has special characteristics of theory and emphasis. Therefore, practice requires attention not only to the fundamental principles of all exercises but also to the features and technical keys of the individual routine being practiced. Likewise, each of the four health qigong routines should also be practiced with emphasis on its particular features. Otherwise, the exercises will lose their core value.

For example, Health Qigong *Wu Qin Xi* emphasizes the imitation of the movement qualities of five animals, while Health Qigong *Liu Zi Jue* emphasizes breathing. During the process of practicing Health Qigong *Liu Zi Jue,* the practitioner should focus mainly on inhaling and exhaling with simple complementary body movements. Furthermore, Health Qigong *Yi Jin Jing* emphasizes the stretching of the sinews and bones, particularly the rotation and flexing of the spine, while Health Qigong *Ba Duan*

Jin emphasizes the exercise of the physical body and regulation of the internal organs, and calls for a focus on the accuracy and aesthetic qualities of the movements.

Practice Hard

Long-term, consistent health qigong practice confers numerous health benefits, but an instructor can at most instruct; it is up to the student to practice. As the ancients said, the teacher introduces the skills, but the practitioner acquires them through hard practice.

In general, practice should progress from simple to complex, easy to difficult, less to more (in intensity and amount). However, greater intensity or energy expenditure does not equate to a better workout. It is not only unnecessary but unproductive to equate "hard practice" with exhaustion or burnout. The standards of what constitutes "hard practice" in health qigong are based on the condition and needs of the individual practitioner.

It is the responsibility of the individual practitioner to determine the appropriate level of intensity, difficulty, and duration of practice, based on their awareness of their own condition. Increase the intensity, difficulty and duration of the practice to the limit of what you feel comfortable with; this is what we call "hard practice". In terms of overall progress, it is better to start with a little practice each day, then increase gradually. The body goes through a process of adapting to practice, as a result of which practicing at greater intensity and duration comes naturally over time. Overdoing it in the beginning will slow things down rather than speed them up, like pulling on a shoot to help it grow. Practitioners who are feeble and ill should take particular care not to wear themselves out with practice, since it may hinder their rehabilitation. The state of the body after practice should be comfortable and pleasant, not tired or exhausted, or at most no more than can be recovered from by the next day. The formula for managing practice load is thus simple: if you feel tired, rest, or reduce the intensity or duration of practice.

The refinement of technique also progresses organically and at a self-determined rate. It is better to allow this process to happen over time, without pushing, than to strive to have perfect technique, which creates tension and nervousness. For example, in "Tiger Springing on Its Prey" of Health Qigong *Yi Jin Iing*, the hands and all ten fingers need to be pressed against the ground. This posture can be approached gradually by first allowing the knees to bend and pressing the hands against the ground beside the legs, then moving comfortably into the full posture over time. The "horse stance" in Health Qigong *Ba Duan Jin* is another posture that is often difficult for beginners; when practicing the horse stance, it is better to begin in a higher posed stance and gradually sink the body down as comfort allows than to begin in a very low posed stance and overload the body's capacity.

The foundation of "hard practice" is to firmly grasp the details, keys and patterns of each routine, understanding the effect of each movement. Watch, ask, think, read, and learn continuously about qigong. Practice and watch others practice, compare and analyze, recognize the strengths and weaknesses of other practitioners, be aware of your own weakness and avoid making the same mistakes as others. This is the way to ensure further advancement.

Be Mindful of the Warming Up and Closing Movements

Warming up serves the purpose of preparing the practitioners mentally and physiologically for qigong practice. It is a transition state crucial for the exercise to have the intended benefits. Warm-up exercises should not be done mindlessly or in a hurry, and certainly shouldn't be ignored.

The warming up exercise stimulates every range of motion, every body part and every internal organ, gradually improving the sensitivity of the nervous system and the flexibility and coordination of the limbs. It helps the brain to eliminate distracting thoughts and paves the way for achieving tranquility. This type of overall stimulation helps the different parts of the body to awaken and activate, as well as relaxes the entire body, all of which assists the flow of blood and qi, preparing the body for the main exercises. Warming up exercises should be done with full attention, and of course, their duration and intensity should be determined by the needs and capacity of each individual practitioner, leaving plenty of energy available for the main exercise. There is no point to being exhausted from the warm-up.

The ending/closing movements are likewise quite simple but very important. They make up a critical component of practice.

The first purpose of the ending movements is to consolidate the effects of the practice session and help them settle in; also, since the different exercises focus on the training of different parts of the body, the ending movements are an opportunity to re-balance the qi and blood throughout the body. The second purpose of the ending movements is to allow the body to return to the normal state gradually. The process of practice has been described as "hard farming", and the ending movements are the process of harvesting and storing all the harvest. If the ending movements are neglected, qi and blood will not be unified and settled, over time causing stagnation and deficiency. The promise of a strong, healthy body will not be realized and, in contrast, health may even be harmed.

Lest we till without reaping, the ending movements should always be practiced with full attention and followed by a period of rest.

Improve Theoretical Understanding and Cultivate Scientific Awareness

Health qigong has several distinct features as a health practice. In the relationship between mind and body, it emphasizes the role of the mind in guiding the body. In all kinds of qigong practices, it is always essential to minimize mental activities, to retract your mind from all affairs of daily life, such as work and study. Focus all your attention on the practice. This is the foundation and the first essential feature of health qigong. The second is that in the relationship between humans and nature, it emphasizes humans coordinating with the changes in nature to form harmony. The third is that in the relationship between individuals and society, it emphasizes harmony within society and moral cultivation, leading to the saying, "*morality is the mother of practice* (德为功之母)".

More than simply a way to overcome sickness and promote health, health qigong is a way of comprehensive cultivation of physique, personality, behaviors, and morality that relates to all aspects of each individual's life. Health qigong is deeply rooted in traditional Chinese culture, drawing from its diverse wisdom, including Confucianism, Taoism, Buddhism, martial arts, and medicine.

Therefore, despite the relative simplicity of its movements, health qigong is a systematic exercise guided by a rich and comprehensive underlying theoretical framework. Since its inception, it has been written that one key to practicing qigong well is to strengthen one's theoretical knowledge; otherwise, it is no different from any other physical exercise. One way to put this teaching into practice is to read the classics and become acquainted with the guiding principles derived from traditional Chinese culture, to in other words absorb the essence and discard the dross of the cultural context from which qigong derives its meaning. Only by understanding the big picture of health qigong as a source of philosophical insight can we truly practice it well.

Create Good Conditions for Practice

Success requires not will alone but also certain conditions, which have been classified as *fa* (right method, 法), *lü* (positive companionship, 侣), *cai* (sufficient resources, 财), and *di* (right setting, 地). Consider starting a business as an example. Choosing the business field and learning the way of doing it would be *fa*, the support of family and friends would be *lü*, cai would be business capital, and the location of the business would be *di*. Likewise, the practice of health qigong requires favorable objective conditions.

There are many different forms and styles of qigong practice, which should be selected from according to the practitioner's condition and needs. The four health qigong routines are good choices. The routines were compiled by experts from the Chinese Health Qigong Association after being tested by numerous practitioners, proving that the routines are simple, reliable and effective. Many experts have contributed to the teaching and systematization of health qigong, ensuring that the routines embody the best practice approaches.

Second, find pleasant, like-minded companions to practice with. Good companionship not only makes practice more enjoyable but also improves the learning process, promotes advancement, and raises the level of benefit gained from practice. Joining a practice group can be a good way to gain these benefits, as long as it is a group that you fit in well with.

To spend money on health is a popular way of life, since many of us are capable of spending more money for better health. The practice of health qigong requires little, but a certain amount of money input is still required for such things as taking classes and buying learning materials.

The ideal practice setting for health qigong is a quiet, comfortable place with fresh air, and regular practice environments should be maintained jointly by the practitioners. A proper practice setting helps to quiet the mind, promote progress and accelerate the effects of practice. Crowded, noisy, and windy places, such as banks of rivers, balconies, rooftops, and windy hillsides, are less than ideal.

Chapter 10

The Scientific Approach to Health Qigong Practice

Previous sections talk about the principles of health qigong practice and how to obtain optimal benefits from one's own practice. This section uses examples from the four Health Qigong routines to introduce the scientific approach to Health Qigong practice, in order to facilitate an easier learning process.

Techniques for Health Qigong *Yi Jin Jing*

Proper Application of Strength

One of the features of Health Qigong *Yi Jin Jing* is extended movements that stretch the sinews by exercising the bones. These movements stretch muscles, tendons, ligaments, joints and joint capsules, enhancing the strength and flexibility of the soft tissues and improving the functioning and activities of the hard tissues.

For example, when practicing the movement "Nine Ghosts Drawing Sabers", put your hands respectively on BL 9 (*yù zhěn*, 玉枕) behind the head and *jiā jǐ* (夹脊) on the back of the trunk, and move the arms like a bird flapping its wings, in order to expand and sink the chest alternately, which enhances the strength and flexibility of the chest muscles. For aged people with declined respiratory function or patients with chronic breathing difficulties, this movement can help to relieve their symptoms and improve their quality of life.

It is best not to use full strength in producing the movements. The specifications for the movements of Health Qigong *Yi Jin Jing* are that the movements should combine hardness and softness and be substantial and non-substantial at the same time. Achieving softness within hardness and hardness within softness requires using appropriate strength in practicing.

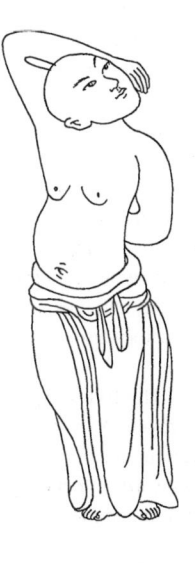

Therefore, only 70% of your strength should be used in the most forceful movements in Health Qigong *Yi Jin Jing*, such as: pushing the palms outward in "Wei Tuo Presenting the Pestle 2", pushing the arms upward in "Wei Tuo Presenting the Pestle 3", pulling the arms inward and outward in "Pulling Nine Cows by Their Tails", pushing the palms forward in "Showing Talons and Spreading Wings", and pressing the palms downward and raising the hands upward in "Sinking the Three Bodily Zones". The force applied in these movements must not be stiff and rigid, otherwise, adverse effects and discomfort could result, especially for elderly practitioners, as well as those with weaker physiques or with chronic shoulder diseases (e.g., frozen shoulder).

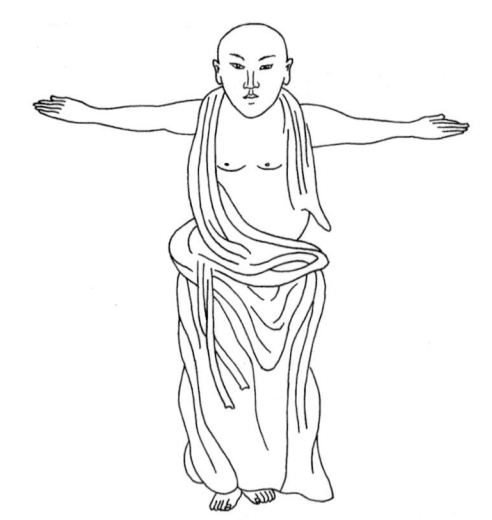

Natural Breathing

The main breathing technique in Health Qigong *Yi Jin Jing* is natural breathing. Regular abdominal breathing, reverse abdominal breathing, and other intentional breathing techniques are not used in the practice.

Both regular and reverse abdominal breathing depend on the contraction and relaxation of the abdominal muscles for a rhythmic inward and outward movement of the abdomen. Heath Qigong *Yi Jin Jing* focuses on the training of the sinews and bones through body movements and still postures. These movements should be combined with natural breathing, because intentionally combining abdominal breathing with them could cause discomfort.

In some cases, practitioners with a solid foundation of qigong practice may grasp the movements and techniques quickly. However, after getting used to the movements, a handful of these practitioners are likely to feel dizzy while practicing. It has been discovered that this often happens when practitioners who are accustomed to combining breathing techniques with body movements, a common approach in many other qigong forms, apply this approach to *Yi Jin Jing* practice by habit. Although they may notice a lack of coordination of their breath and movements, they tend to believe it is because they are not yet used to the practice, and thus insist on continuing the approach. The forced breath regulation in this approach leads to respiratory disorders which result in insufficient oxygen supply, the root cause of their dizziness.

The following is an example of improper breath regulation causing the mentioned result: In the movement "Showing Talons and Spreading Wings", stand the palms in front of LU 2 (*yún mén*, 云门), the acupoints on the chest (please refer to the diagram in the appendix), while expanding the shoulders backward. In natural breathing the human chest cavity is initially expanded, the abdominal muscles are relaxed and move with the chest, and negative pressure within the lungs is created. In regular abdominal breathing, the abdomen is relaxed while inhaling, the diaphragm moves downward, the lower abdomen bulges and the chest muscles are relaxed and in passive movement. The activities of the chest and abdominal muscles in these two breathing methods are different, and improper application of breathing technique could cause the movement and breathing to be uncoordinated, and also lead to respiration disorders and diminish the beneficial effects of practice.

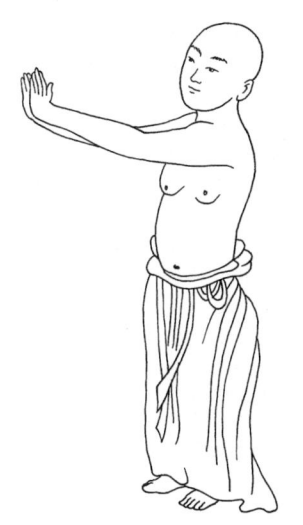

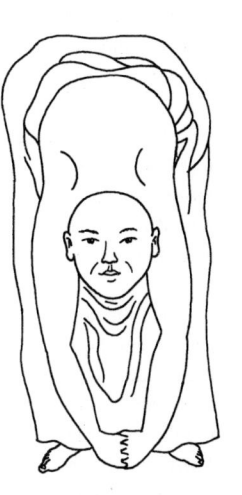

As another example, in the posture of "Swinging the Tail" (upper body bent forward with the head and tailbone raised, chest expanded and waist pulled downward), it is very difficult for a person to use either regular or reverse abdominal breathing while turning the head and swinging the tailbone in such a posture.

Therefore, one should breathe naturally when practicing Health Qigong *Yi Jin Jing*. Give up the intention to inhale and exhale in any specific way. Simply let the chest expand and shrink naturally following the body movements, and the inspiratory capacity and respiratory rate will follow the body movement and be adjusted spontaneously. This will prevent breathing difficulties, shortness of breath and other similar symptoms caused by a disassociation of body movements and breathing. Moreover, natural breathing can help practitioners to relax their bodies and calm their minds, to gradually improve posture and movement for the purpose of improving physical constitution and cultivating health.

Concentration of the Mind

The most important feature of Health Qigong *Yi Jin Jing* is to transform sinews and bones, and thus it is a practice focusing on body movement. Although it is neither a practice of mind guiding body nor a practice of mind in an active role and body in passive role, conscious activities are critical in practicing the movements.

Health qigong practitioners all should know that one of the fundamental requirements in health qigong practice is to control mental and conscious activities throughout practice to avoid being affected by distracting thoughts. At the same time, one should regulate the mind to keep it from being influenced by external distractions. Observe your inner desires and restlessness caused by external distractions, and you can control and constrain them. As a fundamental requirement in the practice of Health Qigong *Yi Jin Jing*, it is important to concentrate and focus; do not let your mind run away.

Mind regulation issues were prevalent when health qigong was taught to college students in traditional sports majors. The students, usually earnest and concentrated in the beginning, often begin to show difficulty in concentration around the sixth or seventh movement. When running through the complete routine, some students display a floating mind and distracted attention after the first third of the routine.

There are at least two possible reasons for this effect. The first is the mental fatigue resulting from continued use of attention in the learning process, and the students' lack of available willpower to overcome the feeling of fatigue. The second reason is that these students usually concentrate on very dynamic practice routines, such as free combat (*sanda*), martial arts (*wushu*), Chinese wrestling, and others. The students thus have been habituated with a dynamic mindset, and this, combined with the fact that they were also practicing dynamic exercises at the same time that they were learning health qigong, may have made it more difficult than normal for them to concentrate.

When ordinary people learn and practice Health Qigong *Yi Jin Jing*, they also face the same mind regulation issues, including distraction of the attention and a floating mind, especially beginners and those who have pressures in daily life. This is a universal issue faced by all Health Qigong *Yi Jin Jing* practitioners, and can only be overcome by earnest training. It should be understood that the mental activities and body movements are opposing but also unified.

Health Qigong *Yi Jin Jing* is not only a form of health exercise targeted at transforming the sinews and bones by body movements, but it also affects the nervous system by effectively regulating mental activities, which is critical in regulating life activities. Therefore, effective regulation of mental activities is the key and core of the "three regulations" (breath regulation, body regulation and mind regulation) of health qigong practice. There was an old saying that "*Bodhidharma came from the west, bringing with him no word, only the training of the mind* (达摩西来无一字，全凭心意用功夫)". One who neglects mind regulation, fails to concentrate the attention, and has a lot of distracting and floating thoughts is no longer practicing "health" qigong.

Failing to concentrate the attention will affect the results of Health Qigong *Yi Jin Jing*, practice, causing the movements to be rigid and stiff without any softness, or to be soft without any strength, failing to stretch and exercise the bones and sinews, failing to positively influence the motor functioning, the autonomic nervous system, the sympathetic or parasympathetic nervous system, or the nervous-humoral-immune function.

The Opening and Closing Posture of Health Qigong *Wu Qin Xi*

"Ready Position: Adjusting the Breath" and "Convey Qi to *Dantian*" are respectively the opening and closing postures of Health Qigong *Wu Qin Xi*, which are critical in the entire routine. It is impossible to achieve the desired results of practice without a proper beginning and ending to the routine.

Ready Position: Adjusting the Breath

The role of the opening posture in the entire routine is that of spring in the cycle of the four seasons. Spring is when life begins, and everything is starting to grow and full of vitality. The breath exercise in the opening posture helps practitioners to extend the breath to be fine and long, and helps to concentrate the mind and eliminate distracting thoughts in order to enter a peaceful state in harmony with nature.

Many practitioners ignore the preparation before practicing, and don't start to move and pose until the background music starts. This makes it difficult to relax and calm the mind during practice. The correct approach is to get yourself ready for practice and adjust your posture before starting the routine by retracting the abdomen and buttocks, sinking the chest and straightening the back, clearing the mind and eliminating distracting thoughts, containing the mind and concentrating your attention on the elixir field (*dān tián*, 丹田), and entering into the state of a peaceful mind with a relaxed and comfortable body. When the background music begins, start the movements in an easy and comfortable way.

Difficult Points in the Opening Posture

The key movement in this posture is raising and pressing the arms and guiding the qi throughout the body. Raise the arms slowly, rotate the wrists to face the palms upward, pull the fingers together and separate the thumbs from them, relax all the fingers and sink the centers of the palms, let the arms hang apart at the same width as the shoulders, extend the arms forward naturally with the elbows slightly bent, and when the arms reach the height of the chest, draw the hands toward each other with the palms facing inward and the four fingers pointing toward each other; then slowly draw the hands toward acupoint RN 17 (*dàn zhōng*, 膻中) on the chest until about 10cm out, then turn the hands to face the palms downward, sinking the shoulders and elbows and pressing the hands downward to the level of the lower elixir field in the lower abdomen, then relax and let the hands go back to the original position.

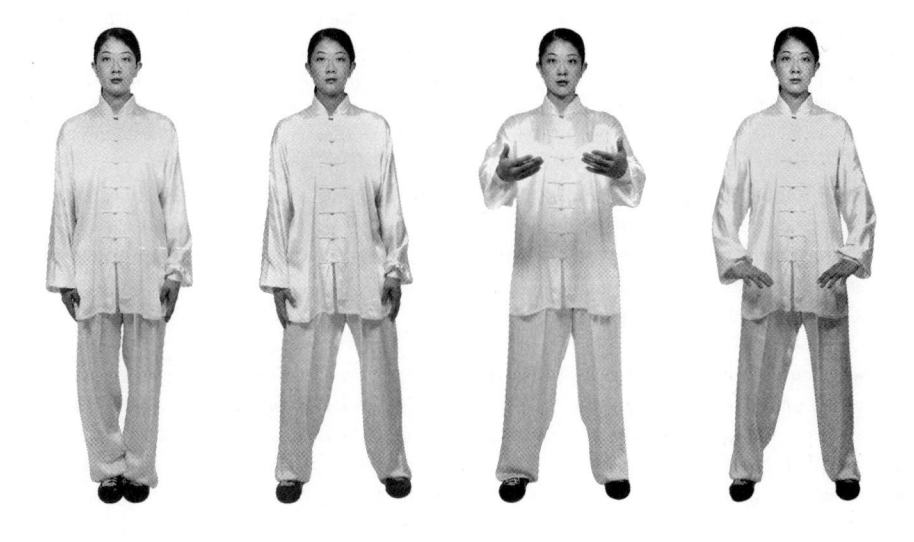

Common Mistakes in the Opening Posture

A common mistake is holding the arms rigid when raising the hands and drawing them toward the chest. The correct approach is to overturn the hands while raising the arms, forming a circular arc with the arms. If the arms cannot move smoothly and form angles comfortably, breathing difficulties can cause the body to become rigid. It is important to enhance your mental awareness of the movement, pay attention to how your arms move and when to draw the hands inward, and also to coordinate the shape of your arms with the breath.

Maintain the correct hand formation, with the thumb separated and the other four fingers together. It is critical to maintain the posture in an easy and comfortable way. Be taught but not rigid, be relaxed but not slacked, enclosing the strength within and manifesting it through the movement.

Maintain the correct body posture. Let the eyes gaze horizontally forward, let the feet be as steady as rocks and the body as firm as a pine tree. The other parts of the body should also be steady and not sway with the arms' movement. Practitioners should adjust the body posture and mental state before proceeding with the movements. Avoid movements of the other parts of the body while moving the arms, such as protruding the buttocks or abdomen, throwing out the chest, or dropping or raising the head.

The "Three Regulations" in the Opening Posture

Mind Regulation: Concentrate on acupoint PC 8 (*láo gōng*, 劳宫) at the centers of the palms while lifting the hands upward, posing the hands as though holding up a big ball of qi which has mass but no physical shape; when the hands reach the height of the chest, turn the palms as though holding a ball of qi, close the hands as though the ball is shrinking, and imagine qi pouring into acupoints RN 17 from the palms; then turn the palms to face downward and press down, imagine the qi pouring into the lower elixir field from the middle elixir field (the region of RN 17). In the entire movement of the opening posture, qi circulates between the centers of the palms and the elixir field, forming an endless loop.

Breath Regulation: The breathing technique in the opening posture is the same as the pattern in the five animal exercises, following the pattern "inhale while ascending and exhale while descending". Inhale while lifting the hands and drawing the hands inward, and exhale while pressing the hands downward. The breath should be fine, long, even, deep, and in harmony with the body movements, and calm and quiet instead of fussed and hasty.

Body Regulation: The famous poet Tao Yuan-ming in the Tang Dynasty wrote a poem that said "*Build a cottage in the world of people, yet you would not hear the noise of carts and horses. If asked how you achieve it, keep your heart at a distance and the place will be remote* (结庐在人境，而无车马喧。问君何能而，心远地自偏)." While practicing Health Qigong *Wu Qin Xi*, the practitioners need to "keep the heart at a distance to be remote". In performing the opening posture, one must shut off all external distractions and be in harmony with the environment, in order to become a unity of qi and mind.

Between each exercise, there is a connecting movement to adjust the breath. It requires the practitioner to raise the arms to form a forty five degree angle with the body, palms facing upward, and draw the hands toward RN 17 on the chest: when the hands are level with the chest, the movement becomes the same as the opening posture. The purpose of this connecting movement is to adjust the breathing, relieve fatigue, serve as a buffer between the movements, and to facilitate the change in artistic quality of the movements.

Closing Posture: Convey Qi to *Dantian*

In the closing posture, which guides qi back to the elixir field (*dantian*), raise the hands beside the body until they are above the top of the head (the arms should be in the same vertical plane as the body, and the palms should face upward), then, bend the elbows to bring the palms toward each other to the same distance apart as the shoulders, and straighten the arms; then bend the elbows, and with the palms facing downward press the hands downward slowly to in front of the abdomen. In the entire process, let the eyes gaze horizontally forward, but focus your mind on the palms, keeping the body upright, and following the breathing pattern of "inhale while ascending and exhale while descending".

Practitioners may adjust the range of motion according to their own status. Those who have pain or diseases of the shoulders or back should not force the height the arms raise to, but move according to their own ability and progress step by step. This can prevent disturbance to the unity of mind and breathing caused by forceful movement. Those who have hypertension should also be cautious, since the arm raising motion might cause the qi and blood to rush upward, resulting in dizziness. Therefore, raise the hands to an appropriate height and imagine your qi and blood flowing downward; this will help to lower your blood pressure.

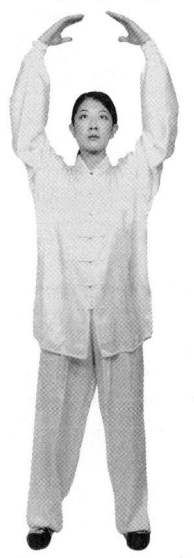

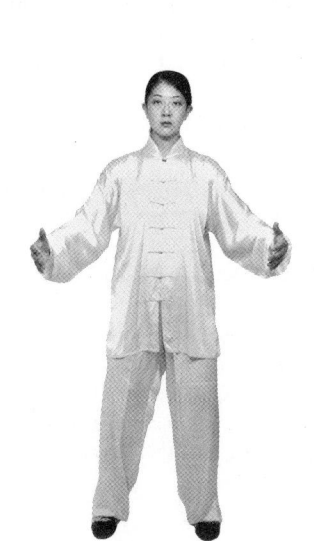

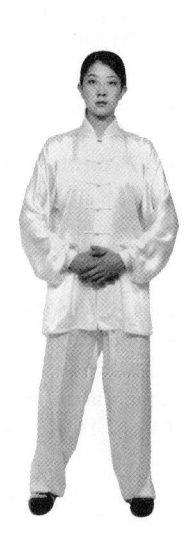

In this movement, raise the arms slowly beside the body, focusing the mind on acupoint PC 8 at the center of the palms; hold the palms as though holding a heavy weight, as though holding the sun or moon, or as though holding a big ball of clear qi from the heaven and earth between the palms; then draw the hands toward each other while raising the arms, shrink and condense the qi ball until finally enclosing it in the two palms above DU 20 (*bǎi huì*, 百会) at the vertex of the head; then press the palms toward the head and pour the qi ball into DU 20; the qi will flow through the upper elixir field, middle elixir field, and finally into the lower elixir field, and circulate throughout the entire body; let the mind follow the flow of qi.

Keep the body upright throughout the movement; do not let the movement of the arms disturb the posture of the body, avoid such defects as leaning the body backward, protruding the abdomen, or dropping or raising the head. Only when the body is posed in an upright position can the qi flow smoothly throughout the body and achieve the desired results.

The traditional Chinese philosophy of "unity of humans and nature" is embodied in the opening and closing postures introduced above. Raise the hands to receive the clear qi from heaven, draw the hands inward to pour the clear qi into the body, press the hands downward to connect the qi with the earth and take in the rich earth qi. Repeat the process again and again and it will lead you into a state of harmony with heaven and earth. Equip yourself with the mind to unite with heaven and earth in practicing, immerse yourself into the surrounding nature, forget where and when you are and unite yourself with all that surrounds you.

Keys and Techniques in Health Qigong *Liu Zi Jue*

Pronunciation, the shape of the mouth and the specification of breath are the unique techniques in Health Qigong *Liu Zi Jue*. They are the key and core of the practice. During practice, the pronunciation should be adjusted continually to get an accurate mouth shape, by which to control the inhalation and exhalation of the breath. Breaths with different fineness, magnitude and techniques have regulative effects on the qi mechanisms of different organs and body parts. This is not only the approach and procedure of Health Qigong *Liu Zi Jue*, but also the objective and effect of it, and therefore needs to be learned and experienced earnestly.

Correct Pronunciation

Liu Zi Jue (The Six Sounds) has been applied and developed extensively in the past in various areas, such as medicine, health cultivation, *wushu* and others. Because of the different understandings of practitioners from these different fields, plus the long history of the practice and the variation of accents in different geographical areas, there are many views and arguments on the sounding of the six sounds in *Liu Zi Jue*. After extensive research, the pronunciation of Chinese *pinyin* was adopted as the official pronunciation, which is critical in the *Liu Zi Jue* techniques. The pronunciation is as follows:

xū (嘘), hē (呵), hū (呼), sī (呬), chuī (吹), xī (嘻)

How to Pronounce the Sounds in *Liu Zi Jue*

According to the studies of experts and the records in qigong, Chinese medicine and phonology documents, the Chinese characters of the six sounds all have " 口 " ("mouth") as radical, and each of these six characters represents a certain state of the human body.

Use the sound xū (嘘) as an example; after finishing a stressful job, we instinctively sigh with a sound similar to "xū —", which helps to release stress and depression and makes us feel relaxed and happy. The effect of it can hardly be achieved if the sigh (i.e. the xū sound) is pronounced precisely according to the pronunciation of the character in mandarin or *pinyin*. The effect of the sound can only be achieved under a particular state of the body by using the specific sounding, mouth shape, and breathing, which is the principle of *Liu Zi Jue*.

Still using the xū (嘘) sound as example, it is created by combining the initial syllable of "x" and the second syllable of "ü", to form the sound "xū" which is short and quick. The "xū" sound in *Liu Zi Jue* should be coordinated with the breath; this means the length of the sound should be as long as the exhalation. If you continue the sound "xū (嘘)", it becomes "ü" instead of "xū (嘘)" at the end.

The same principle is applied to other sounds in the practice. A special note is that the pronunciation of the six sounds is not only based on the sounds of mandarin and *pinyin*; there are specific mouth shapes and breath techniques that induce particular states of the body which are used to fulfill the purpose of health cultivation.

The Volume of Sound

Beginners of Health Qigong *Liu Zi Jue* should pronounce the sound in an audible way, louder in the beginning and lower later on. When getting used to the practice, beginners can also practice in a silent way with the same mouth shape and exhalation technique, achieving the state of "sound with no sound".

Mouth Shape and Tips for the Breathing Technique

Xū (嘘) Sound

Mouth Shape: Part the mouth and teeth slightly, pull the corners of the mouth back to pull the lips flat slightly, leave a gap between the upper and lower molar teeth, let the tip of the tongue stay flat, and withdraw the tongue backward slightly; there should be a gap between each side of the tongue and the molar teeth.

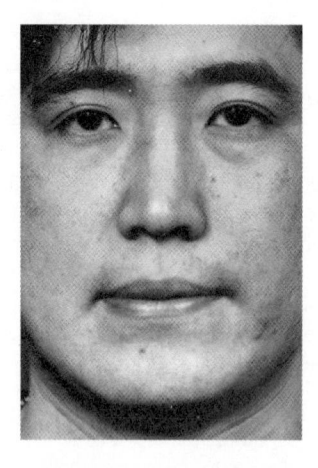

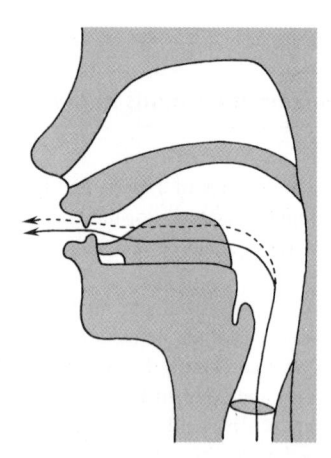

Tips: Part the mouth and teeth slightly to pronounce the syllable "x"; the mouth shape then is the basic mouth shape for this sound; on this basis pull the lips flat slightly to pronounce the syllable "ü".

Feeling the Breath: Maintaining the described mouth shape, first exhale the breath through the slits between the molar teeth and the gaps between the tongue and the teeth, and then through the corners of the mouth. The sound pronounced in such way is very close to the sound "xū".

Though the exhalation needs to be accompanied by sound, the breath becomes very fine with repeated practice, making it difficult to feel its flow and leading to finer and finer sounds. However, this is in accordance with the specifications for breath regulation, that is, to be "even, fine, soft, and long". This same principle is applied to all the other sounds in *Liu Zi Jue*.

Hē (呵) Sound

Mouth Shape: Part the mouth and teeth slightly, draw the tongue backward slightly and push it upward, let the sides of the rear part of the tongue touch the upper molar teeth slightly.

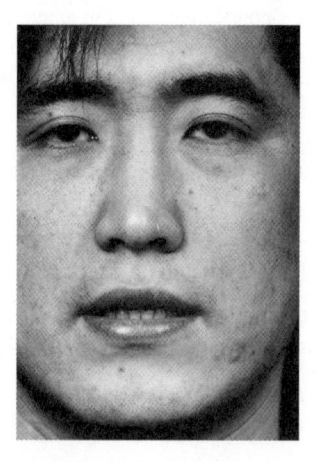

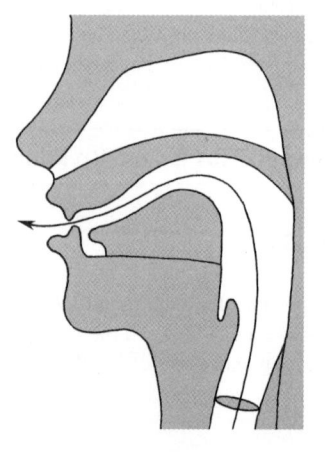

Tips: Part the mouth and teeth slightly and pronounce the syllable "h", which is the basic mouth shape of the hē (呵) sound. Continue to pronounce the syllable "e" on the basis of this mouth shape.

Feeling the Breath: Maintaining the described shape of the mouth, soundlessly exhale the breath. The breath should be exhaled between the surface of the tongue and the upper palate. The sound pronounced in such way is very close to the sound "hē".

Hū (呼) Sound

Mouth Shape: Part the mouth and teeth, form a circle with the lips and protrude it, rolling both sides of the tongue.

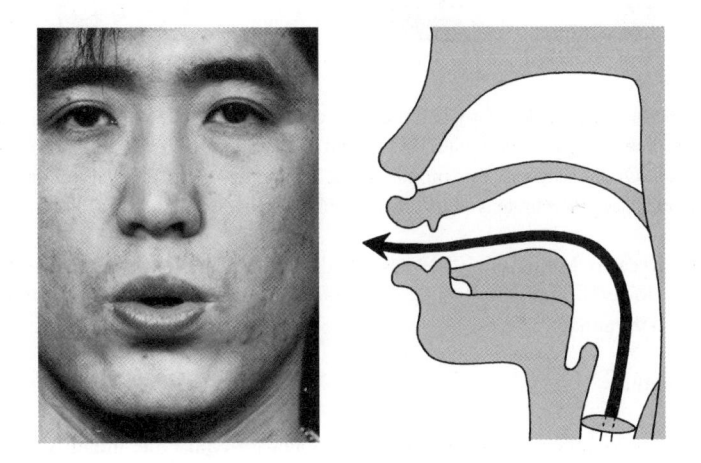

Tips: Form a circle with the lips, protrude it with the lips relaxed, as if blowing out a candle; pronounce the sound of "hū" on the basis of this mouth shape.

Feeling the Breath: Maintaining the described mouth shape, exhale soundlessly; the breath should go through the throat and form a flow in the mouth cavity, then be exhaled slowly through the circle formed by the lips; the sound pronounced by this mouth shape is very close to the sound "hū".

Sī (呬) Sound

Mouth Shape: Mouth parted slightly with the teeth closed, upper front teeth in line with the lower ones; lay the tip of the tongue flat and touch it to the lower teeth gently; pull the corners of the mouth backward slightly.

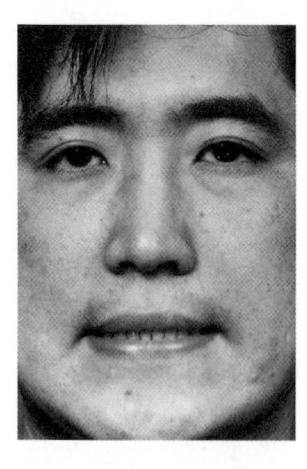

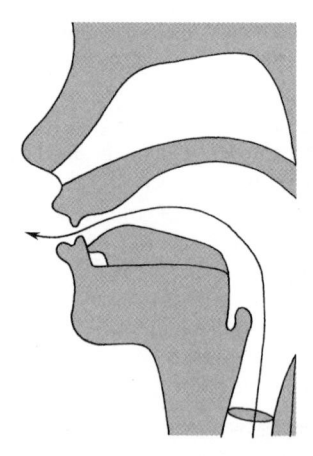

Tips: With the mouth parted slightly and the teeth closed, inhale with a "sī" sound, like a sound you might make when feeling cold in the winter; the mouth shape then is the basic mouth shape for the "sī" sound in *Liu Zi Jue*. On the basis of this mouth shape, exhale instead of inhale and pronounce the "sī" sound. If the pronunciation is accurate, you can feel the vibration and cool feeling of the front teeth.

Feeling the Breath: Maintaining the described mouth shape, exhale soundlessly; the breath should be exhaled slowly through the slits between the front teeth, and the sound pronounced in such a way is very close to the sound "sī".

▪ Chuī (吹) Sound

This is the most complicated one among the six sounds, because the mouth shape is a dynamic one. It is broken down into three steps for easier learning:

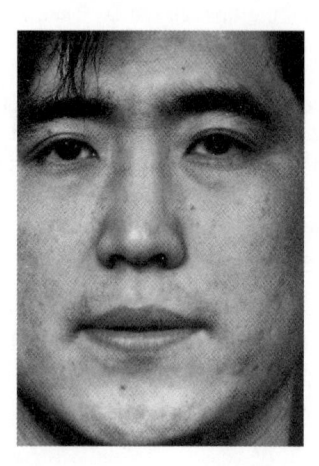

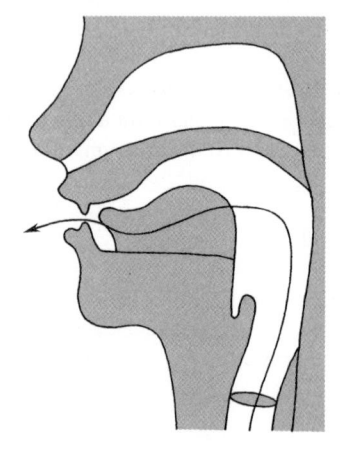

Step 1: Touch the tip of the tongue gently to the inner side of the upper teeth, part the lips and teeth slightly, and make the sound of "ch";

Step 2: Close the parted lips slightly, lay the tip of the tongue flat and make the sound "u";

Step 3: Part the lips again and at the same time touch the tip of the tongue gently to the inner side of the lower teeth, making the sound "i".

The "chuī" sound is formed by linking the three steps together.

Since the mouth shape is dynamic, the breath flow is also full of changes. To summarize, the breath goes through the throat, around the sides of the tongue, then under it, and finally is exhaled between the lips.

Xī (嘻) Sound

Mouth Shape: Lips parted slightly with the teeth closed, upper front teeth in line with the lower ones. Join the molar teeth together as if biting slightly, lay the tip of the tongue flat and touch it gently to the lower teeth; pull the corners of the mouth backward slightly.

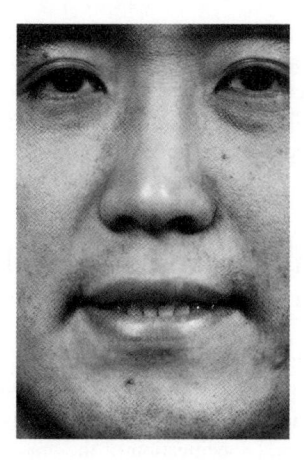

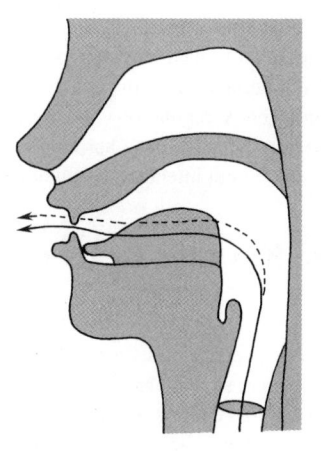

Tips: The mouth shape of the "sī" sound is also the basic mouth shape for the "xī" sound; pull the corners of the mouth backward, and join the molar teeth together as if biting, then exhale and make the sound of "xī".

Feeling the Breath: Maintaining the described mouth shape, exhale soundlessly. The breath should go through the slits of the rear teeth and be exhaled through the corners of the mouth; the sound pronounced in such way is very close to the sound "xī".

About "Breath"

The practice of Health Qigong *Liu Zi Jue* is a direct training of breath, and therefore it is critical to use proper breathing techniques.

There are mainly two breathing techniques in the practice of Health Qigong *Liu Zi Jue*; one is natural breathing, with inhalation and exhalation both through the nose, and the other one is reverse abdominal breathing, with nose inhalation and mouth exhalation. Natural breathing is applied throughout the routine except when pronouncing sounds in exhalation, where reverse abdominal breathing should be applied.

The ancients called one inhalation plus one exhalation "one breath", and thus the technique for adjusting inhalation and exhalation is called "breath regulation", which is a fundamental technique and one of the "three regulations" in qigong practice.

The basic requirement for breath regulation is that the breath be even, fine, soft, long, and deep. Also, the breath should be trained in a step by step way, rather than by learning by rote or seeking for a particular result deliberately. Breath regulation should be built on the foundation of a relaxed but properly posed body (body regulation) and a peaceful mind (mind regulation). Through long term practice, one will naturally achieve the harmony of body, qi, and mind, and achieve an even, fine, soft, long, and deep breath without intentional regulation.

The Keys for Learning and Practicing Health Qigong *Ba Duan Jin*

"Learning" is the process of acquiring knowledge or skills while "practicing" is the process to advance and become more skillful. Hence practice in the process of learning and learn in the process of practicing; the two form an endless process and are complementary to each other. The core of learning and practicing is "approach", including the principle and specification of the practice, as well as the characteristics, keys, requirements, and other aspects. Here we give a brief overall introduction to the Health Qigong *Ba Duan Jin* routine, instead of a detailed explanation of all the aspects.

Health Qigong *Ba Duan Jin* Focuses on the Training of the Body

The standing form of *Ba Duan Jin* (Eight Pieces of Brocade) is an ancient *daoyin* practice. Throughout its one thousand years of development and evolution, regardless of the variation or time period, its focus has always been on the training of the body. Through the movement of the body, it enhances the functioning of the internal organs, frees the channels and collaterals, and harmonizes the qi and blood circulation, for the purpose of strengthening the body and promoting health. The best approach for learning and practicing this routine is to "cultivate the body" to "walk the way of the Tao".

In learning and practicing Health Qigong *Ba Duan Jin*, the technical skill of body movement can be broken down into three stages:

Beginning stage of learning: Start from basic body postures, hand formations and footwork. First gain a general overview of the practice, then take time to practice each of the movements individually. Emphasize the training of particular postures or moves while practicing the typical movements of the routine. You should be able to move in a way that basically matches the specifications of the routine.

Practitioners should work hard on meeting the specifications of the movements, getting hold of the three elements "point, line and shape". "Point" is the starting and ending points of the routine, "line" is the route and procedure of the movements, and "shape" is the shape of the body, including both dynamic movements and still postures. All parts and sections of the routine should be performed clearly and be distinct from one another, and you may pause when performing the routine to make the movements distinguishable. Practitioners should be well aware of the feelings of all body parts. The upper body should be upright and the lower body steady, and the foot formations and footwork, hand formations and handwork should be clearly and accurately performed according to the specifications. People sometimes say "*seek for the square*[34] *first, then the circle*[35] (先求方，后求圆)", which refers to the same principle.

Adaptive stage — becoming more skillful: Correct and improve the movements through repeated practice, in order to be skillful at and master all of them. Pay attention to the shifting of the body weight and balance, and also to the connecting movements. Drive the limb movements by the waist and spine, so as to make the movements soft, slow, fluid, flexible and coherent; the entire body and all the movements should be in harmony.

Advanced stage — enhancing the skills: On the basis of the previous stages, emphasize the elements of relaxation and peace, emptiness and solidity, strength and softness, and internal force in the practice. Practitioners should relax both internally and externally, calm the mind, and concentrate all attention on the practice. The movements should be light and agile, distinct in stretching and contraction, combine emptiness and solidity, and shift properly in every change. Accumulate softness to become strength, integrate strength and softness, and be moderate in relaxation and tightness, emphasizing intention instead of force. Feel the interconnection among the "three regulations" in order to move the body freely, calm the mind, adjust the breath in a spontaneous way, and gradually achieve the unity of the three regulations.

The Exercise of the Spine is the Core of Health Qigong *Ba Duan Jin*

The spine has the function of supporting the body and protecting the internal organs, and is also

---

34. "square" here means "rules"
35. "circle" here means "fully understanding and have one's own way"

the center of human motions, in charge of physical body movements. The spine can be referred to as "the second life line". It is found in clinical studies that spinal disease has become one of the biggest hidden health threats in the 21st century.

The influence of the spine on human health has been taken fully into account in the compilation and creation of Health Qigong *Ba Duan Jin*, and therefore the practice emphasizes the training of the spine. In each and every movement, the internal force is accumulated and initiated from the *jia ji* (the hollow on both sides of the spine and in between the scapulas), and all the motion in this routine is centered around the axis of the spine. The *du mai*[36] passes through the spine and connects with all the other channels and collaterals, and the acupuncture points on the bladder channel on both sides of the spine connect with the internal organs directly, and therefore a slight movement of the spine activates the movement of the entire body. In Health Qigong *Ba Duan Jin*, you should seize the motion pattern of the spine and the pattern of internal force application, which is the essence of this practice.

To help practitioners understand the role of the spine, here we list the keys to all the movements below:

Ready Position: In "Ready Position" and all the other ascending, descending and standing movements in the routine, the spine should move as a whole but in a flexible way, as if it is a string of beads, with force transmitted throughout the entire spine.

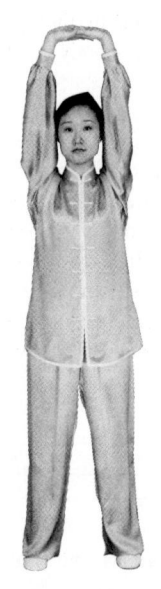

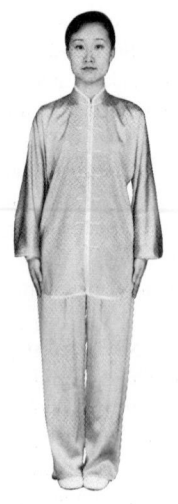

Holding the Hands High with Palms Up to Regulate the Internal Organs: Pushing the palms upward, straighten and stretch the spine, transmitting the force upward to PC 8 (*láo gōng*, 劳宫) at the center of the palms and to *jia ji* on the back.

---

36. *Du mai* — one of the extraordinary channels in the human body; the concept of channels and collaterals is a critical part of TCM theories.

Posing as an Archer Shooting Both Left- and-Right-Handed: Cross the wrists and relax the *jia ji*, straighten the spine and transmit the force to the *jia ji* while posing as an archer.

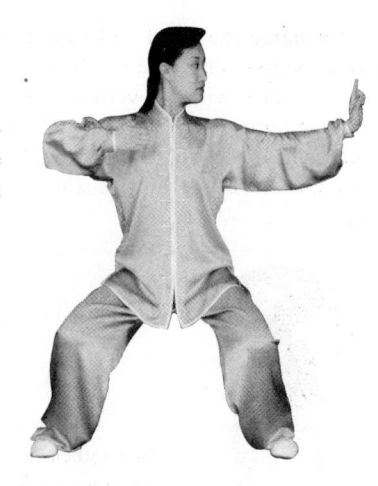

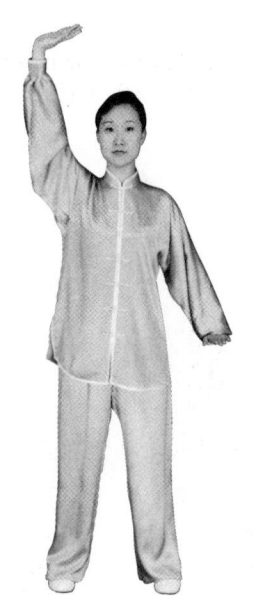

Holding One Arm Aloft to Regulate the Functions of the Spleen and Stomach: Part the palms, extend them upward and downward respectively and stretch, with internal force reaching PC 8 at the center of the palms and the *jia ji*.

Looking Backwards to Prevent Sickness and Strain: Holding the palms as specified, push the vertex of the head upward and straighten the spine, pull the shoulders backward and look back, with the force reaching the *jia ji*.

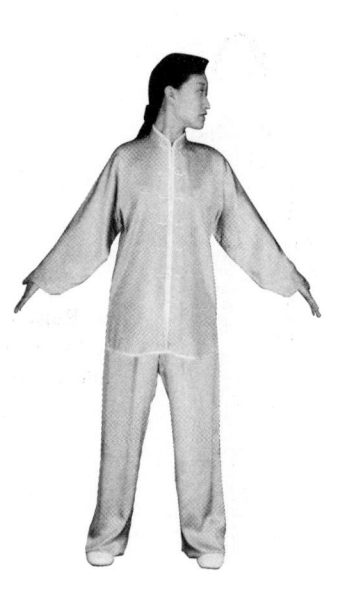

Swinging the Head and Lowering the Body to Relieve Stress: Press the hands on the legs while in a horse stance, with the vertex pushing upward and the spine straightened; stretch the spine and waist while leaning the body sideward and bending the body forward, and twist the tailbone while rotating the upper body.

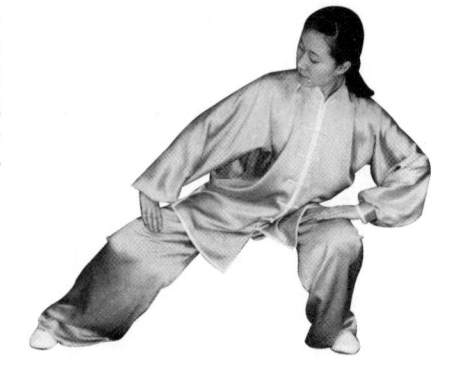

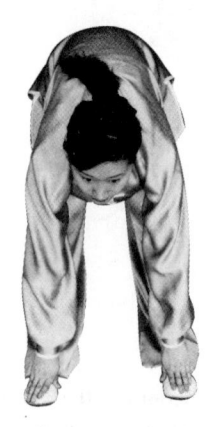

Moving the Hands down the Back and Legs and Touching the Feet to Strengthen the Kidneys: Stretch the spine while straightening the body, relax the spine while bending the body forward.

Thrusting the Fists and Making the Eyes Glare to Enhance Strength: Push the vertex upward and straighten the spine while squatting into a horse stance; twist the spine while thrusting the fists out.

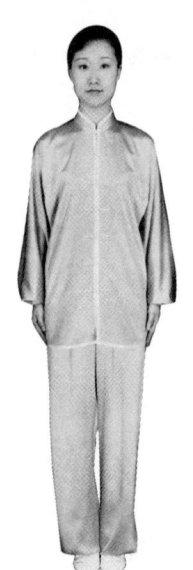

Raising and Lowering the Heels to Cure Diseases: Stretch the vertebrae one by one while raising the heels, feel the vibration between the vertebrae while lowering the heels.

Closing Form: Relax the spine, return to the original position, and end the routine.

The "internal force" here does not to mean to use strength or to exert force. The body becomes stiff while using strength, and qi and blood cannot circulate smoothly. Therefore, "internal force" should be explained as applying intention instead of applying strength; it is a compound of *shen* (mind), *yi* (intention) and qi.

The "Ready Position" is Critical in Health Qigong *Ba Duan Jin*

The "Ready Position" in Health Qigong *Ba Duan Jin* is a popular movement; it is called "*tai ji*" stance" in the *tai jiquan* circle, and called "three-round posture" or "ball-holding posture" in the qigong circle. The posture is rich in content, and it is the first choice for qigong and *tai ji quan* practice, and thus referred to as "the first stance of posture practice".

There are three reasons why it is designed as the first movement of Health Qigong *Ba Duan Jin*.

1) As a basic posture, that is, the physical body in a still state. It is the most typical posture in qigong practice; the practitioner should push the vertex upward, straighten the neck and spine, sink the shoulders and elbows; the chest should be empty and the abdomen solid, and the entire body should be in an upright and comfortable position.

2) As a basic movement, that is, the most basic and rhythmic movement. The "Ready Position" appears repeatedly between all the sections and movements, and is critical in connecting the entire routine. Mastering this movement helps the practitioner to advance.

3) As a basic skill, that is, the essential quality and ability for qigong practice. By practicing "Ready Position", practitioners can be trained in all aspects, as it covers all the principles, keys and elements of this routine, which are critical in mastering the skills and enhancing the effects of practice.

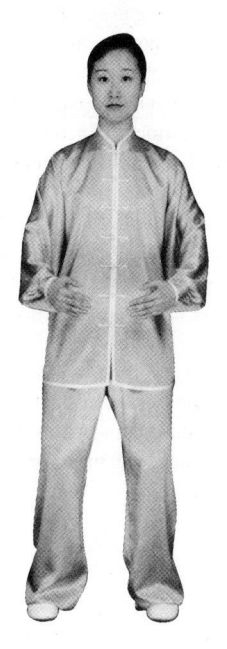

The above factors explain the importance of "Ready Position" in Health Qigong *Ba Duan Jin*. It not only prepares the body and mind for practicing the routine, but is also a critical part of the routine, and therefore should be strongly emphasized.

There are many approaches for practicing "Ready Position"; here we give a brief introduction. Practitioners should focus on improving body shape in the beginning stage, correcting mistakes and improving the skills through repeated practice, until they become automatic. Do not interrupt your own breath, but let it be natural, concentrating your mind on regulating the body shape. For example, practice "Ready Position" as a basic exercise, but understand that such practice serves to promote mastery of the entire routine. Practitioners should strengthen their physique, which is essential for qigong practice, solve the technical issues in the routine, and harmonize the relationship between intention (mind), qi, and body.

The first stage is to "*steel the mind, labor the sinews and bones* (苦其心志，劳其筋骨)". This means overcoming the muscle soreness, joint numbness, and clumsy movements in posture practice. This stage is called "*force conversion* (换劲)". It usually takes around three weeks to go through this stage. The first week is sometimes painful, the body starts to loosen up in the second week, and the limbs and waist become strong after three weeks and begin to feel comfortable.

The second stage is based on the foundation of the first stage, and seeks to relax and calm both the mind and body, also known as creating relaxation and tranquility. Relaxation is the prerequisite; relax the entire body thoroughly from head to feet, from inside to outside, and down to each pore on your skin. Tranquility means to get rid of distracting thoughts, "*seize the heart-ape, and tie the mind-horse* (收猿心，栓意马)[37]", trying to be calm and peaceful and concentrate on practicing. There are different levels of relaxation and tranquility, which are difficult to achieve within a short term; it may take years or decades for a practitioner to settle the issue, if it happens at all. It is remarkable if a practitioner can achieve totally the state mentioned above.

In the third stage, with the deepening of relaxation and tranquility, the breath will be slower, and the internal qi activated, as practitioners slowly enter into a peaceful state of cultivation. Be "indifferent" in such a state, but not "empty", do not be greedy for the state you are in and seek it at an appropriate time. Long term practice will increase physical strength, refresh the mind, and cheer you up.

One thing to pay attention to is that, in this routine, it is not suggested to drop the eyelids while practicing, and certainly not to shut the eyelids. Also, practice with a proper intensity. Stop immediately and make adjustments if any adverse symptoms appear during practice, including palpitation, shortness of breath, dizziness, or tremors.

---

37. Heart-ape & mind-horse: In original Chinese, these are used to describe the restless and hesitant mind, and distracting thoughts; in other words, a mind that is jumping like an ape or running like a horse.

Chapter 11
Notes for Health Qigong Practice

We have used a lot of space to introduce the principles of scientific health qigong practice, and to generalize how to learn and practice the four health qigong routines. In this section, we will emphasize some of these issues in greater detail, to help practitioners learn and practice health qigong in the best way possible.

Grasping the Scientific Approach

A scientific approach is essential for any kind of sport, for without it, adverse consequences are likely to result. The same is true for health qigong. Health qigong trains "mind", "qi", and "body" as a unity, and thus needs to be practiced in a more cautious way. If you train the "mind", "qi", and "body" in an appropriate way, your health will be promoted. In contrast, practicing inappropriately will lead to nothing beneficial being achieved, or even to harm.

Therefore, practitioners must earnestly learn the techniques from the beginning. Also, one must maintain a good physical and mental state in order to avoid detours, and to achieve maximum results with minimal effort.

The Purpose of Practice

A purpose is the target or result you want to achieve. A proper purpose is necessary to ensure the beneficial effects of practice. The purpose of health qigong practice should be to strengthen the body, cultivate health, prolong life, and promote rehabilitation. It is improper to practice for personal profit alone or merely to seek out as a novelty.

Qigong practice is not mysterious, nor is it either simple or complicated, nor vulgar. Practitioners should be fully intentional in practicing, be determined, practice earnestly with perseverance, and proceed step by step, rather than practicing in fits and starts.

Practitioners should also seek the cultivation of personality and morality in daily life; a light heart and a generous, noble and open mind will keep you happy and peaceful, and help to avoid the distractions caused by burdensome emotions and desires.

Preparation before Practice

The basic requirement of qigong practice is to help the brain enter into a state of "tranquility". However, we often have distracting thoughts, and may find it difficult to concentrate and calm the mind. Therefore, practitioners should prepare in advance and get ready for practice by eliminating distracting factors as much as possible, to ensure a smooth delivery.

- Ease your mind and emotions before practicing. If your emotions are unsteady or irritated, a lot of distracting thoughts will be the result, causing a restless mind and irregular breathing, which will affect the outcome of practice. If you experience extremes of emotions such as joy, rage, sadness, grief, panic, fear, or others, take a walk someplace with fresh air, and don't go back to practicing until your mind is calmed and released from the emotions.
- Do not wear tight clothing. Practicing with appropriate clothing lets your body be comfortable and allows for smooth blood circulation. Accessories, such as belts, watches, or bracelets, should be avoided if they are too tight, as well as tight shoe laces or garters. Also, do not wear high heels or tight shoes or other hindering attachments.
- Relieve the bladder and bowels before practicing, and cease any intense physical activities long enough beforehand to stabilize the body and mind.
- Before beginning to practice, become fully warmed up by doing preparation exercises or stretching exercises. This helps to bring your body into the practice state and prevent sports injuries.
- Choose an appropriate place for practicing. The environment should be clean and quiet (avoid external disturbances and agitations) with fresh air. Do not practice outdoors under severe weather (such as rain, fog, wind, etc.). Practice indoors instead, but do not practice when there is thunder or lightning. Do not practice when you are very hungry, very full, too tired, or after drinking alcohol. Eating too much hinders the circulation of qi and blood, it will be difficult to relax and to concentrate the mind when you are too hungry or too tired, and alcohol disturbs the qi mechanism. Do not practice where the air is severely polluted, such as places with a heavy chemical odor, or damp places smelling of rotten substances or garbage.

Paying Attention to the Movements

There are specific meanings and effects for each technical detail of the routines (covering mental, qi and physical aspects). The outcome of practice is greatly affected by how well a practitioner masters the techniques. Proper techniques promote the circulation of qi and blood, while inaccurate techniques hinder the circulation of qi and blood.

Therefore, practitioners should earnestly strive to experience these effects, through repeat practice in strict accordance with the keys and specifications of the routines, which help to promote the positive effects of health qigong practice.

Do not correct mistaken movements and techniques while performing a complete routine, but rather check and adjust mistakes in casual practice. Otherwise, the peaceful and concentrated mental state will be disturbed, affecting the effectiveness of practice.

Practice according to Your Own Condition

Younger people have a stronger learning ability and receptivity, but they are more impatient. Speed is a relative concept, and skill is accumulated gradually. Do not jump to another step when you are not ready; such haste will make progress come slowly. Make sure you understand every detail thoroughly, perfect your skills through continual and repeated practice, and progress will be fast. The practice of health qigong is not merely an exercise for the physical body, but also a training for the mind. Haste will weaken the training of the mind, and you will fail to achieve the target of cultivating both body and mind by exercising haste.

The flexibility of middle-aged and aged practitioners has declined, and thus they should increase the intensity of practice gradually. Blindly increasing the difficulty in haste, ignoring your own physical condition and adaptability, will easily result in muscle strain and increase the burden on the heart and the consumption of essence and qi.

There are no strict rules for the practice time of health qigong, and practitioners may arrange practice according to their own schedules, but it is suggested to practice every day. Female practitioners in menstruation should not practice for too long, and should temporarily suspend routines involving heavy intensity.

Effects Determined by Details

Many details of practice are ignored by practitioners, but are important factors determining the outcome of practice.
- Do not speak while practicing. If there is an emergency, close the practice by collecting the qi into the elixir field. Avoid chatting.
- Do not be anxious for physiological responses. Some responses might appear in practice, such as feelings of heat, cold, soreness, numbness, swelling, or beating of the muscles. Do not pay too much attention to these responses, and do not seek for any responses deliberately; neither be happy nor afraid once they appear, simply let them be and neglect them, and then they will fade away. Of course, ask your tutor for help if serious or drastic responses arise.
- Keep your body warm if practicing in cold and damp weather. If you sweat during practice, change clothes immediately afterward. Do not take a cold shower or bath immediately after practicing.
- Avoid practicing while tired. If you feel tired, close the practice session and rest. Avoid being too tired in daily life to avoid deficiency-consumption and internal damage. *"excessive standing impairs the bones, excessive walking impairs the sinews, excessive use of the eyes impairs the*

blood (久立伤骨、久行伤筋、久视伤血)", thus one should work and take rest alternately. Practitioners should pay special attention to their sex lives to avoid impairment caused by sexual indulgence, especially for people in poor health or patients of certain diseases (hypertension, heart diseases, tuberculosis, liver diseases, kidney diseases, ulcers, neurasthenia and others). Overindulgent sex is an impairment to health.

➢ Close the routine properly when finished practicing. After finishing, take a walk for a few minutes. Do not sit or lie still immediately after practicing, and do not eat or drink until your qi and blood have settled.

➢ Qigong is a practice of health cultivation. As such, practitioners should combine it with other health cultivating activities in daily life, like avoiding bad habits such as smoking and drinking, having a regular schedule, and getting sufficient nutrition, physical exercise, and rest.

Health qigong provides excellent rehabilitation for many diseases, but it is not the panacea to heal all illness, and not everybody can practice it. For some diseases, especially acute diseases such as acute appendicitis, you should go to the hospital immediately. You may start to practice health qigong for rehabilitation after relieving the acute symptoms. Patients of chronic diseases should continue proper medications while avoiding drug abuse. Unconscious patients, patients with bleeding, mental illness, hysteria, acute diseases, or severe functional failure of the heart, brain, lung, liver, and kidney should not practice health qigong, and those with acute infectious diseases, such as atypical pneumonia and the infectious period of hepatitis, should not participate in group practice.

Chapter 12

Issues in Health Qigong Practice

Motion and Stillness

Many practitioners have concerns about the issues of "motion" and "stillness" in practice. We have touched upon the issue in the chapter "The Principles of Health Qigong Practice" and we will talk more about it here.

The Differentiation and Unity of "Motion" and "Stillness"

Motion and stillness are the two aspects of movement, but they are at the same time united. "Motion" is absolute and "stillness" is relative. Everything in the universe is developed from unceasing motion and changes.

The same philosophy is in the overall characteristic and inherent pattern of health qigong. Motion includes the motion of the physical body and the activities of the mind; while stillness covers the calmness of the mind and the stillness of the physical body.

Motion is yang and stillness is yin. Yin and yang interact with each other; they are interdependent, and the dynamic equilibrium of yin and yang can be achieved through reciprocal growth and decline, and inter-transformation between the two. In the same way, motion and stillness in health qigong are an indivisible organic entity, and the two promote each other.

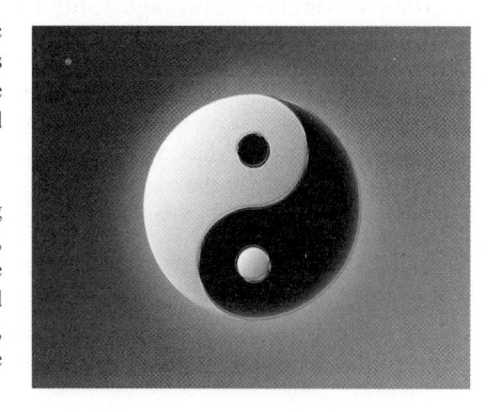

"Stillness" within "Motion"

"Motion" here is the bending, stretching, rotation, turning, opening, closing, and other movements of the physical body under the influence of consciousness. "Stillness" is the seeming pauses in the movements, while actually the internal force is still running and the muscles are still extending or contracting. The motion and stillness of the body cannot be divided in an absolute way; they are compatible and inter-transformable.

For example, in "Nine Ghosts Drawing Sabers" of Health Qigong *Yi Jin Jing*, the movement pauses (i.e., is still) when expanding the chest in an elbow-bending posture. The chest and arms are not relaxed or completely still at the pause; in contrast, you should pull the scapulas inward toward each other to stretch all the connected sinews and bones. And when you pause while pulling the bent elbows toward each other and sinking the chest, the muscles should work in a contrary way.

Another example, in "Holding the Hands High with the Palms Up to Regulate the Internal Organs" of Health Qigong *Ba Duan Jin*: cross the hands in front of the abdomen, and lift them to in front of the chest; the body is still in this procedure except for the upper limbs. When the arms rotate inward to push upward, all parts of the arms should move in a consecutive way. When expanding the chest and abdomen by extending the arms, pull your chin inward slowly, and let your eyes gaze forward. The shoulders and arms are seemingly still in this entire process, but the muscles are actually stretching and extending.

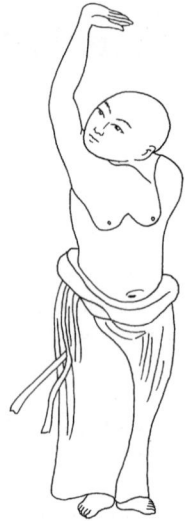

The same compatibility and inter-transformation theory of "motion" and "stillness" can be applied to all other routines and movements.

"Motion" Manifested through "Stillness"

The activities of the mind are the various mental activities preceeding body movements, such as intention and concentration. They also refer to mental states with relatively strong psychological activities. Peace of mind is the stillness of mental activities, a quiet and calm mind and consciousness, or a mental state with relatively weak psychological activities preceding movement. Peace of mind and consciousness is only a primary state of tranquility; the more advanced levels of tranquility are not a subject we will discuss in this book.

In health qigong practice, it is required to concentrate all your mind and consciousness on body movements, to unite the body and mind, and avoid any other mental and psychological activities. That is, avoid thoughts and ideas irrelevant to what you are practicing, such as distracting thoughts, drifting consciousness and imaginings. Quiet your consciousness in the harmony of body and mind; intention is not required here.

The nature of yin and yang are relative; there is nothing that is absolute yin or absolute yang. Therefore, mind regulation techniques (e.g. concentrate the attention on a certain part of body) need to be applied in some movements, in order to enhance the effect of the movement and to adjust the qi flow. However, these mental techniques should be used in an appropriate way and not overused; simply concentrate the mind or focus it on a certain target.

In "Plucking Stars" of Health Qigong *Yi Jin Jing*, it is required to gaze at the raised palm while concentrating your mind on DU 4 (*mìng mén*, 命门) on the back of the waist. In the various exercises of Health Qigong *Wu Qin Xi*, practitioners are required to consciously imitate the charm of the animals. Also, practitioners should concentrate on the elixir field in the closing forms of all four health qigong routines. These are all examples of some of the mental activities specified in health qigong practice.

Overall, the mind regulation activities in health qigong practice are to manifest through the physical body. Do not guide the movement by your mind but keep your mind in a relatively "still" state, letting it follow your movement as reflex, which manifests as activity of mind. Unite the body and mind in such a way, let the mind and qi follow each other, and you will achieve the result of strengthening the body and enhancing health.

"Relaxation" and "Tension"

Application of "Relaxation" and "Tension"

"Relaxation" and "tension" could be manifested both as activities of the muscles and activities of the mind.

The variation of muscular strength and mental activity intensity in practice is based on the traditional philosophy of yin and yang, that the external movements and internal mental activities are perfectly combined. The variation of force and the continual force application in different movements could bring a certain amount of energetic stimulation to the corresponding body parts, which has the effect of relieving stagnation and muscle adhesion, lubricating the joints, strengthening the bones and sinews, and improving the overall physical constitution. A relaxed mind enables the body to move in ease, comfortably and gracefully, for the purpose of harmonizing qi and blood, freeing the channels and collaterals, and cultivating the body and mind.

"Relaxation" and "Tension" in Body Movements

The "relaxation" and "tension" of the body refers to "relaxed" and "tense" ways of moving.

Relaxed movement involves the muscles working at minimum strength. That is, the body joints can extend, bend and move in many ways when there is zero resistance from the muscles. In the process of making a movement, we need to exert force and tension with the muscles for large-scale extension or contraction of the joints; this is tense movement. In such a process, the extended muscles become tense due to stretching or resistance, and other synergistic muscles become tense as well.

"Softness" in *daoyin* movement is "relaxation". "Relaxation" is a relative state instead of an absolute state; it is not a sluggish state without any strength. "Relaxation" is how the connecting movements act to transfer from one still movement gradually to another one, in a relatively slow and easy process without any sudden force or momentary relaxation.

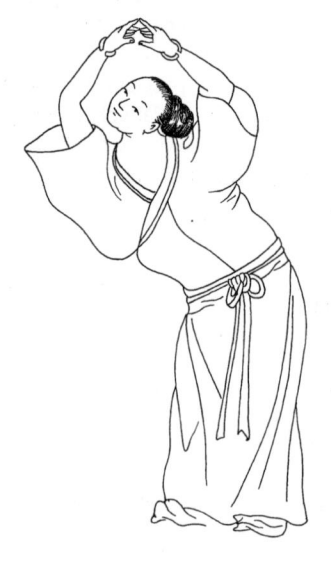

As an example, take "Holding the Hands High with the Palms Up to Regulate the Internal Organs" of Health Qigong *Ba Duan Jin*; the movement of the arms dropping down after raising up; in "Pulling Nine Cows by Their Tails" of Health Qigong *Yi Jin Jing*; the pulling back, rotation and pulling outward of the arms in Health Qigong *Liu Zi Jue*; and the rising, descending, opening, closing, pushing aside, and gathering back of the hands; all these body movements have the characteristics of light, soft, smooth and slow. The relaxation of the muscles after tension helps to relax and calm the mind, regulate the nervous system's activities, and improve and balance the physiological functions of the various system and organs.

"Hardness" is the "tense" movement of exerting force. Examples are the movement of expanding the chest and stretching the shoulders in "Showing Talons and Spreading Wings" of Health Qigong *Yi Jin Jing*, and the movement of clenching the fists while lifting and lowering the hands in "Tiger Exercise" of Health Qigong *Wu Qin Xi*. The muscles in these movements should be in a relatively tense state and exert a proper amount of force; do not apply strength forcefully. Absolute force exertion is "hardness without softness"; such a force is brutal and will cause the movements to be rigid. The various body joints cannot be fully extended under such a state, as well as the muscles and other soft tissues. It is in violation of the traditional principle of the coexistence and united motion of yin and yang.

The transition between "tension" and "relaxation", or "hardness" and "softness" of movement is a gradual process of inner transformation. The force that extends the joints is developed gradually from a weaker force to a stronger force in a relaxed and soft way; the force that contracts the joints is gradually transformed from "tense" or "hard" to "relaxed" or "soft".

For example, the movement that imitates a deer running in "Deer Exercise" of Health Qigong *Wu Qin Xi* should be slow, relaxed, soft, light and comfortable. When the shoulders, back and arms extend to form a transverse arc, and the body trunk and spine stretch to form a vertical arc, the movement pauses for a moment. However, the muscles and joints are not slack in the pause, and the breathing continues, rather than being restricted by the tension of the body. The force transforms continually, giving the movement strength but not rigidity, relaxation but not sluggishness. Integrating both yin and yang in the movement prevents the adverse results caused by extremes.

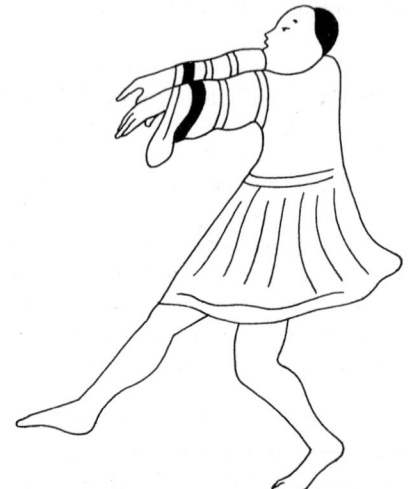

The "Relaxation" and "Tension" of the Mind

When the body is moving, mental activities and their intensity (such as intention, concentration, attention, consciousness, etc.) reflect the "relaxation" or "tension" of the mind. The "relaxation" of the mind, in routine practice, refers to the weakening of the intention to guide body movement consciously, or the weakening of the attention on certain body parts. The "tension" of the mind, in routine practice, refers to the intensification of mental activities.

"Relaxation" of the mind means not only to relax and calm the mind, but also to be indifferent and weaken the intention to guide the body's movements, avoiding deliberate intention and obsession. The intensification of mental and conscious activities is just a relatively stronger state compared to the peaceful mind, indifferent to movement.

For example, in "Sinking the Three Bodily Zones" of Health Qigong *Yi Jin Jing*, you should imagine holding something heavy while pressing the palms down and lifting them up, but the intensity of the visualization should be mild. In "Showing Talons and Spreading Wings", push the palms forward as though pushing a mountain, but the force must not be rigid and brutal.

Also, in practicing Health Qigong *Wu Qin Xi*, both the body and mind should relax and concentrate on nothing but the mind itself, adopting the moods of how the five animals play and frolic. On the basis of maintaining appropriate body postures and movements, relax all the muscles as much as possible, be natural and comfortable instead of stiff, rigid, tight, or sluggish.

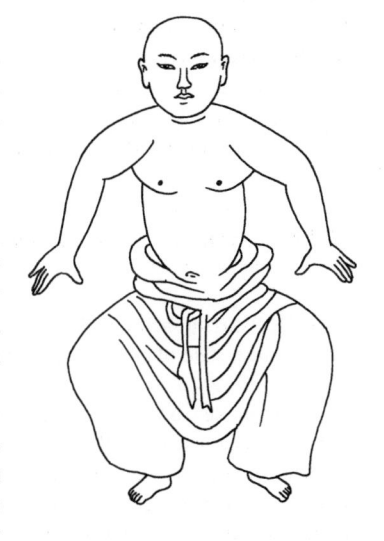

In Health Qigong *Ba Duan Jin*, the archer posture with horse stance in "Posing as an Archer Shooting Both Left-and Right-Handed", the raising hand in "Holding One Arm Aloft to Regulate the Functions of the Spleen and Stomach", and the punching and clenching fist in "Thrusting the Fists and Making the Eyes Glare to Enhance Strength" use tension, but the "tension" in these movements is relatively momentary compared to the "relaxation" throughout the entire practice.

In other words, the force applied in health qigong movements and the "tension" of mind and body should be appropriate; the momentary forces should be intentional but also indifferent. This helps to balance the yin and yang aspects of the movements and promotes health. It also prevents harm caused by mental stress and tension.

The "tension" of the body and the "relaxation" of the mind are relative, and should be coordinated and unified. When a body part is exerting force or when the muscles and joints are in a relatively tense state, the mind should relax; in addition, other muscles and parts of the body must not be tense and should be fully relaxed. This can prevent the reverse flow of internal qi caused by tension, exercising the body without toiling the mind, cultivating both together.

"Stirring Sensations"

The common subjective feelings after practicing health qigong are ease of emotions, a pleasurable and refreshing mind, and a comfortable and relaxed feeling of the entire body. Some practitioners may have special feelings of warmth, coolness, muscle pulsing, lightness and/or floating, heaviness and/or sinking, relaxation, tightening, streaming of heat, or electric current. The ancients classified these sensations into: stirring (*dong*, 动), itching (*yang*, 痒), coolness (*liang*, 凉), warmth (*nuan*, 暖), lightness (*qing*, 轻), heaviness (*zhong*, 重), roughness (*se*, 涩), smoothness (*hua*, 滑), and also dropping (*diao*, 掉), leaning (*yi*, 猗), coldness (*leng*, 冷), heat (*re*, 热), floating (*fu*, 浮), sinking (*chen*, 沉), hardness (*jian*, 坚), and softness (*ruan*, 软). In traditional qigong practice, all of these are referred to as "stirring sensations" or "stirring feelings".

The Concept of "Stirring Sensations"

The "stirring sensations" appearing in practice are normal phenomena; they are part of the physiological state of practice and usually disappear after closing the routine.

Stirring sensations may appear as one sensation or several sensations at the same time, or sometimes as sensations other than those recorded or described. These sensations usually start as faint feelings, and the frequency and intensity may increase and then disappear gradually, as the practitioner becomes more proficient. The process of appearance and disappearance of "stirring sensations" is that of the internal qi being adjusted and yin and yang balancing themselves within the body. It signifies the physiological functioning of the body in adjustment and improvement.

However, you must not deliberately pursue the various "stirring sensations". It is harmful to both physical and mental health, interrupting relaxation and tranquility. For example, if you feel your body is "light" during practice, this is a comfortable and normal sensation, but if you try to capture the sensation deliberately or try to reinforce the sensation intentionally, your mind will be tempted by these intentions, resulting in brain excitement, making it difficult to relax both the body and mind and enter into the health qigong state of awareness, diminishing the beneficial effects of practice.

How to Overcome "Stirring Sensations"

One of the positive effects of practice is a joyful mind and a comfortable body. The appearance of "stirring sensations" is neither a good sign nor a bad sign, and should not be a cause for celebration or alarm. The phenomenon is not caused by pathological hallucinations, thought disorders (delusions), disturbances of consciousness (trances), or psychological disorders, and is certainly not a sign of being "possessed". If you feel "cool" in a certain part of the body, the feeling may not be as desirable and comfortable as the feeling of "warmth", and it might be an awkward feeling. Without a proper understanding of the sensations, fear and anxiety could arise, which would hinder the relaxed and tranquil state of qigong practice and thus the resulting outcome. The practitioner's daily life might even be affected by such fears in extreme cases.

Do not subjectively judge the "stirring sensations" to decide whether or not they are normal, and do not pursue or resist the sensations deliberately. Be indifferent toward the phenomenon and do not let your mind and attention be distracted, but continue your practice and daily life as usual. As for the sensations, let them be and do not interrupt, rather let them come and go as they are.

Problems Caused by Improper Practice

If you do not follow the principles of qigong practice, if you are anxious for success or practice with improper approaches, abnormal psychological and physiological changes could be caused, resulting in a variety of strange feelings which are not "stirring sensations". These need to be paid attention to and corrected for. For example, for a practitioner who has a disease of the neck, shoulders, waist or legs, performing body movements in a forceful way could induce aseptic inflammation, resulting in pain; those who have cervical disease may display dizziness, a lack of energy, or limb numbness if trying to perform large movements, because of the anxiety for success; for patients with hypertension, the same mistaken approach could cause a rise in blood pressure.

Disorders caused by improper practice could become a psychological burden for practitioners, affecting daily diet and sleep patterns, and eventually harming the health.

If you cannot distinguish a "stirring sensation" from a symptom of an existing or induced disease, we suggest stopping the practice first. Analyze your own practice, check for any abnormalities or mistakes, and adjust your approach according to the analysis. Receive a medical check-up and seek treatment if necessary, and return to practice when the issue has been resolved.

Group Practice and Individual Practice

Group practice refers to a number of health qigong practitioners gathering and forming a stable group, practicing together based on a specific schedule and location. Individual practice refers to practicing by oneself individually.

Benefits of Group Practice

Studies of sports psychology have shown that sports help to improve character flaws, and that different kinds of sports have different influences on the practitioners.

Each practitioner has a unique personal character, but when a group of practitioners gather together, they can help improve each other's psychological and mental states through mutual learning, communication, and assistance, especially for those who are introverted, unsociable, eccentric, or otherwise not so good with people.

Persistence in participating in group practice will strengthen a practitioner's vitality and spirit of cooperation with others, gradually improving personality. Those who are impulsive and easily irritated or who have difficulty calming down can enhance their ability of self-control through the positive external influence of the group and the regulating practice of health qigong. Therefore, group practice is helpful for improving and regulating the psychological and mental state of practitioners.

Benefits of Individual Practice

For long-term practitioners, regular group practice might sometimes be interrupted by different factors, such as the weather. Sudden breaks might become very uncomfortable for those who are used to practicing routinely. At such times, it is helpful to continue the practice by yourself at home or in any other suitable place.

For those who cannot participate in group practice, which may be due to a variety of reasons, it is beneficial to practice at home or in any other suitable place. Practitioners have different health conditions, family backgrounds, and levels of mental stress and work pressure. If one insists on participating in group practice by disregarding personal limitations, health can hardly be promoted, and in contrast the family harmony could be broken, causing conflicts and bringing negative influences to both body and mind.

Integrating Group Practice and Individual Practice

Group practice and individual practice have different advantages, but neither is absolutely superior to the other. In group practice practitioners can communicate, learn from each other, and complement each other, helping one another to improve together. However, the discipline of group practice needs to be channeled into individual practice for practitioners to continue to advance.

People who cannot participate in group practice can learn from others' experiences through books or videos, partly attaining the effect of group practice. However, the accuracy of postures and movements learned through this approach is low. Therefore, you should learn first from experienced tutors, and then use books and videos as learning aids, and communicate with other practitioners to exchange experiences and ideas. Practicing only by yourself can hardly guarantee the accuracy and persistence of practice, much less the positive effects.

Practice Where a Certified Health Qigong Tutor is Available

If you are a beginner, practice where a certified health qigong tutor is available. A certified or experienced tutor can guide practitioners in both skills and theories, helping them to get hold of the keys of movements, correct their mistakes on time, and develop a daily life pattern following the philosophy of health qigong.

There will usually be a group of practitioners learning from a certified tutor, creating a harmonious environment of group practice regardless of the different backgrounds of the practitioners. Such an environment is ideal for practicing. Long term practice with such a group will lead to mutual understanding among the practitioners and a collective sense of honor, which helps the members to encourage each other and overcome laziness. Practitioners can learn more, share more, avoid detours, get hold of the techniques and skills in a much faster way, and achieve better results through practicing in such an environment.

However, avoid personality worship of the tutor, or blindly believing and following; these will hinder the positive effects of practice and the cultivation of body and mind.

Practicing a Single Routine or Practicing All the Routines Together

Each health qigong routine has its own characteristics. They differ in techniques, movements, keys and style, but all of them emphasize body movements, apply mild mental techniques and natural breathing, and share some common technical features. You may combine the practice of different routines for complementary results; this approach has proven effective for many practitioners in China.

Body Movements in Common

Traditional qigong theories hold that proper body movements can resist aging.

The practice of all the health qigong routines is mainly manifested through body movements. Besides the movements of the limbs and body trunk, the all-directional movement of the spine is very critical. All of the health qigong routines emphasize the bending, extending, rotation, turning, stretching and contraction of the spine, activating the movements of the body and limbs by the action of the spine. The typical examples are "Tiger Springing on Its Prey", "Black Dragon Displaying Its Claws" and "Swinging the Tail" in Health Qigong *Yi Jin Jing*; "Tiger Exercise—Seizing the Prey", "Deer Exercise—Colliding with the Antlers" and "Monkey Exercise—Picking Fruit" in Health Qigong *Wu Qin Xi*; the "*Xu* Exercise" and "*Si* Exercise" of Health Qigong *Liu Zi Jue*; and "Swinging the Head and Lowering the Body to Relieve Stress" and "Moving the Hands Down the Back and Legs and Touching the Feet to Strengthen the Kidneys" in Health Qigong *Ba Duan Jin*.

The health qigong routines also emphasize the movement of the peripheral joints at the distal limbs, manifested as different hand formations and movements, and as how the toes grip the floor. The exercise of the spine enhances the functioning of the spinal joints, driving the functioning of the internal organs and stimulating the spinal cord and nerve root extended from the spine, so as to enhance and improve the physiological functions of the body. Most of the other physical exercises focus on the training of large joints and large muscle groups; the peripheral joints, small muscles, small ligaments and other peripheral soft tissues are often ignored in other forms of exercise, while the training of these body parts in health qigong can lead the movements of the big joints and big muscle groups. The training of peripheral joints in health qigong enhances the coordination between nerves in the brain and the activities of the peripheral joints, as well as the spontaneous regulation of the peripheral nerves. This improves peripheral blood circulation, lowers blood pressure, reduces cardiac load, stimulates the channels and collaterals on the limbs, and promotes the circulation of qi and blood of the internal organs.

Qi and Blood Circulation and Breathing Techniques in Common

The mental guidance of internal qi circulation is not required in health qigong practice as in other forms of qigong. In health qigong practice, the circulation of qi and blood and the regulation of the breath are guided by body movements in a natural and automatic way.

In Health Qigong *Yi Jin Jing*, practitioners are instructed to relax, calm and contain the mind, and avoid concentrating the attention on a certain point or a certain part of the body, but instead allowing it to move as the body moves, change as the posture changes, uniting the body and mind and allowing them to follow each other. Coordinate the breath with the body movements, and let the chest expand or shrink naturally. Cultivation of health is achieved through naturalness.

In Health Qigong *Wu Qin Xi*, it is required to "*guide externally and lead internally, body relaxed with mind fulfilled* (外导内引，形松意充)". "Guide externally" means to move the body in a way imitating the animal movements; "lead internally" means to lead the internal qi movement by external body movements; "body relaxed" means to keep all the muscles relaxed while maintaining accurate body postures, being comfortable and natural, neither stiff nor weak; "mind fulfilled" means to move and pose in accordance with the charm of the five animals, letting the mind and qi follow each other and letting the qi run through the entire body. Do not adjust or hold the breath deliberately; breathe easily, peacefully, and naturally according to the different postures and different applications of force.

Health Qigong *Liu Zi Jue* emphasizes the combination of intention and easy, slow, smooth and flexible movements, applying intention to physical shape in a mild way. Relaxing the body and keeping it natural will help to regulate and optimize the qi mechanism. Apply only the slightest intention to the breath and do not bulge or shrink your abdomen deliberately.

In Health Qigong *Ba Duan Jin*, it is required to ease your mind: "*concentrate as though not concentrating, exist as though barely existing* (似守非守，绵绵若存)". Qi will circulate within the body, following mind and body if the two are in harmony. Be natural in breathing, neither ignore nor subsidize it, and do not breathe forcefully.

There are inherent patterns of how the qi and blood circulate within the channels and collaterals, and of the breathing and qi mechanism. "*The way (Tao/Dao) follows nature* (道法自然)" is a basic principle of qigong practice. Therefore, it is better not to deliberately intervene in inherent patterns, such as intentionally changing, promoting or restricting the circulation of qi and blood or of the respiratory mechanism. Otherwise, disorders of qi and blood circulation or of breathing could easily be caused, resulting in what are called "deviations".

Proficiency with a Single Routine or with All Routines

From the perspective of technical aspects and the effects of practice, the different health qigong routines are basically the same. They all require extended movements, and the movements of the body and limbs should connect and run together smoothly and fluidly. All of the routines emphasize the keys of combining motion and stillness and relaxation and tension, so as to harmonize the circulation of qi and blood and the respiratory mechanism. The routines are all based on the laws of nature, and targeted at strengthening the body, freeing the channels and collaterals, harmonizing the qi and blood, balancing the internal organs, and promoting health and rehabilitation through relaxed, harmonious, natural, and soft body movements.

Yet each of the routines has its own characteristics, creating slight differences between them, such as the intensity of practice. Therefore, it is suggested that practitioners master one routine first, and then on the foundation of that one learn and practice the other routines, since all of their principles are consistent with each other. Practitioners can decide the number of routines and the time to practice based on their own condition, so as to optimize the results of practice according to physical strength.

Chapter 13
Health Qigong Testimonials

In order to give the health qigong enthusiast a clear idea of the results possible by learning of other peoples' experiences, we provide excerpts from the Health Qigong Magazine, sponsored by the Chinese Health Qigong Association.

"I am 76 this year, and retired from a government office. Due to a lack of exercise, I have suffered from high blood pressure and heart trouble, and often feel dizzy. After retiring, I began exercising. At the beginning, I walked ten miles every day on foot, but I felt tired and the effects were not good.

Two years ago, I saw lots of old people practicing Qigong in Yanjing Park in Tangshan. I took part in it without any high expectations. After practicing for some time, I felt better. Now, my legs can move flexibly, and I seldom feel dizzy. To my great joy, my old illnesses have been cured and my physical exam stats have reached the normal index. When I come across friends, they all praise me for my good health and do not believe I am nearly 80 years old. My biggest understanding is that one must persevere in practicing health qigong. So far, I have practiced it for many years, and except when the weather is bad, I often do it outdoors. As time goes by, I believe I can become healthier than ever before.

Liu Yong-ping
Tang Shan, Hebei, China

I am 68 this year, a retired teacher from Hai La Er Zheng Yang street primary school. I often feel dizzy and have suffered from headaches and high blood pressure. My hypertension is between 150 and 180 Pa; the low pressure is between 90 and 110 Pa. I had to take medicine at the same time every day, but the efficacy was not good.

The health qigong I practiced was *Yi Jin Jing* and *Ba Duan Jin*. After learning and practicing for some time, I felt much better and my high blood pressure was alleviated, so I become even more interested in practicing health qigong. I insist on practicing it one hour a day. Because I have become much stronger than I was before, I began to walk one hour every morning and ride for 40 to 60 minutes every afternoon. The inflammation in my left shoulder has gone. Now the hypertension has lowered to between 120 and 140 Pa, and the low pressure is 80 to 90 Pa, a nearly normal index.

Through practicing health qigong, I have become strong in body, happy in mind, and sharp in thinking, and there is no trouble in eating, falling asleep or walking. Many comrades saw me and asked how I kept such good health. "Because I practice health qigong", I said happily.

Li Gui-ying
Inner Mongolia, China

I have practiced the five-animal exercises for two years. Now although I am old, I still can straighten my back, squat, and stand up flexibly. I have benefited a lot from practicing health qigong. Therefore I have a better understanding of the sentence—"the true meaning of life lies in taking exercise". This also firms my belief in practicing health qigong. In order to keep good health and have happy remaining years, and also for carrying forward Chinese traditional culture, I will keep practicing health qigong for my whole life.

Zhang Ruo-zhen
Jiangsu, China

My wife, Ruo-zhen, is a retired primary school teacher. She is 61 this year. Some friends recommend Health Qigong *Wu Qin Xi* to her two years ago. She has benefited a lot from it.

Since she was middle-aged, she had been suffering from rheumatoid heart trouble which caused mitral stenosis and inflicted serious damage on her health. After one operation, she had gotten a little better but often caught cold, and thus the quality of her life was not high. So she began to practice the Five-animal Exercises after retiring. Since then her body condition has changed a lot. Now she looks good and the original symptoms of her disease have gone. Her immunity to colds has become strong. This makes all of us feel happy for her.

Because of her good health, she is happy and does not get irritated, suspicious, or self-abased easily. It was the 40th anniversary of our marriage in April 2005. She invited me to take some wedding photos and told me that it was not a privilege for young people only but also good for the aged to have a taste of its delicacy. She became sociable and interested in everything. Last year, she went to the University of the Aged.

Her changes in body and mind have made my wife have all sorts of positive feelings. She is thankful to be practicing Health Qigong—*Wu Qin Xi*. When I told her that I was going to practice health qigong, she became very excited. Now we have more than ten old friends practicing health qigong. They also made a well-received performance of the activity held by the Wuxi Qigong Association.

Chen Fa-gen
Jiangsu, China

Zhang Yao-ming, a 71 year old retired worker, said happily, "For two years I have insisted on practicing health qigong everyday, and now I am stronger than before." Mr. Ji, another retired worker who was in the same working unit as Mr. Zhang said, "I always caught cold and went to the hospital for physical exams frequently up to a year ago. After practicing health qigong, I seldom catch cold or go to the hospital. When my comrades see me, they always praise me for my good health." Mrs. Yan, a retired office worker said excitedly, "I have benefited a lot from the *Yi Jin Jing* Exercises. Now my original illness symptoms have gone. I can sleep well and I have a much slimmer figure than before."

Hou Xi-rong
Jiangsu, China

I have benefited a lot from practicing *Wu Qin Xi* in the last two years. During the early years, because of over working, I suffered a lot from the ache in my lumbar vertebra, cervical vertebra, shoulder, and knee. After practicing, I can move flexibly. What's more, it has exerted a favorable influence on my temperament and helped me get rid of the burdens weighing on my mind. After I retired, I left the familiar surroundings and felt nobody cared about me, so it was easy to become irritated and sorrowful. However, when I took part in the group exercise, I made lots of friends. We practice together, learn from each other, and provide mutual encouragement, so I feel as happy as before.

Dong Cui-di

Practicing *Liu Zi Jue* has made me strong and kept me from getting sick in the last two years. Although I am already 70 years old, people always think I am no more than 50 years old.

I was an athlete and basketball player before and suffered from knee-joint inflammation. It was hard for me to squat down and stand up.

After practicing *Liu Zi Jue*, I can squat down and stand up flexibly. Besides that, the practitioners in the Health Qigong Station are friendly; we can exchange our opinions freely. The music of *Liu Zi Jue* is soft, gentle, and classic, which also makes me feel calm and pleasant.

The method of practicing *Liu Zi Jue* is easy to learn and master. It is based on the unique pronunciations of the six characters: "Xu", "He", "Hu", "Si", "Chui", and "Xi", which correspond with the liver, the heart, spleen, lungs, kidneys, and three visceral cavities of the internal organs respectively, to regulate the circulation of blood and the vital energy, to improve the functions of the internal organs, to strengthen the bones and joints, and to promote good health. The aged and people who are sick and weak are best suited to practice it. Many friends have already benefited a lot from it.

Xu Guo-cheng
Henan, China

I am 76 years old, a retired officer of the Xinhua Bookstore in Haidian District. Before that, I worked at Beijing Xinhua Bookstore. The reason for my retirement was my poor health. I have suffered from gastric ulcers, deafness, hernia, hypertrophy of the prostate, and so on. What's more, I was vexed about my serious diabetes. In 1984, I was almost desperate, for my uric sugar reached four "plus" and my blood sugar was beyond 200. Because my family has a medical history of cancer, I got gastric carcinoma in November last year, and my stomach has been resected three quarters.

Because the requirements of the actions of practicing the *Liu Zi Jue* are easy, soft and coherent, I chose it to build my body. Now, every morning, I attend the group exercise for half an hour in the park and practice by myself at home in the afternoon and evening. To choose the right time to practice is also very important, especially for patients with a condition like mine. I often practice after meals to consume the sugar in my body. Now *Liu Zi Jue* has become a part of my life.

Insisting on practicing *Liu Zi Jue* has lots of advantages. For example, because of my diabetes and stomach-resection, I often feel tired. But now all of these uncomfortable feelings have gone. I can climb to the fifth stair at one breath carrying twenty Jin (a unit of weight equal to a half kilogram). My other feelings, such as dry mouth and dry eyes, have also disappeared. My blood sugar has also come down and now I do not need to take medicine everyday. I am also able to hear better.

Dictated by An Jie
Recorded by Wang Jian-jun

My name is Chen Baodi and I am 57 years old this year. Since I joined work, my health was not good. For several years I had to go to the hospital for frequent physical exams. After being examined by many traditional Chinese and Western medicine experts, the diagnosis was kidney failure and cervical vertebra disease. I often felt tired yet could not fall asleep, and did not have an appetite. I had to take An Ding medicine to help me fall asleep. The medical care fee was a heavy burden to my family. From 2003 to 2004, accompanied by my husband, we had been to five big hospitals for exams with little effect.

During the spring festival of 2004, when my husband and I went for a walk in Xihui Park, we found more than ten people practicing a kind of Qigong, but we didn't know the name of it. After having a chat with them, we knew the name of the qigong they practiced was Health Qigong *Liu Zi Jue*, initiated and advocated by the State Physical Cultural and Sports Commission. The instructor there told me that the *Liu Zi Jue* was scientific and I should have a try at it. The next day, I went to the practice site early in the morning and learned from the instructor carefully. Since then, I buried myself in practicing and have never stopped. Now, I have an appetite and can fall asleep quickly. Many relatives admire my good health. Some friends who noticed my changes in body and mind began to practice *Liu Zi Jue* last year.

Chen Bao-di
Jiangsu, China

My name is Zhang Huizhen. Although I am 76, I am still in excellent health, and my neighbors always praise me for my vigorous and energetic condition. For many years I have insisted on doing exercises and being broad-minded. After practicing Health Qigong *Ba Duan Jin*, I am much stronger than before.

When I was young, life conditions were hard. I had to over-work to support the whole family. As I became older and older, my physical condition became worse and worse. I had an accident in 1989 when a bus stopped suddenly and I fell down from the seat. This resulted in a fractured back vertebra and dislocation of the pelvic cavity bones. Although the injuries were treated and healed, I have suffered from the secondary effects.

In the latter half of 2003, my neighbor told me that Health Qigong *Ba Duan Jin* would suit me to practice and invited me to go to the health qigong station in the park with her. There in the station, the instructor taught me carefully. I felt comfortable after learning and practicing; the actions are soft and the method is easy to learn. So I decided to practice it regularly.

It has been two years since I began to practice *Ba Duan Jin*. Now I am immune to the cold in winter, and my original aches have gone. In my opinion, aged people should choose their prefered exercises to do and exercise regularly. As for myself, I will insist on practicing *Ba Duan Jin* and realizing the dream of "five generations under the same roof".

Zhang Huizhen
Jiangxi, China

I am 69 years old and have benefited a lot from practicing Health Qigong *Ba Duan Jin*. I had suffered from high blood pressure and joint inflammation before I practiced *Ba Duan Jin*. Now I am stronger and full of vigor. And I can do all the housework by myself, which lightens the burden of my children. My friends often joke with me that I am like a woman of only 49 years. The health qigong makes me look younger, and I am very happy about it. My family members all support me to continue practicing *Ba Duan Jin*.

Zhou Yu-qing (a retired worker)

I am 90 years old. Because of the hard life conditions of the old society, my health was not good at all. I suffered a lot from being hard of hearing and dim-sighted as well as cholecystitis, cholelithiasis, heart disease, a sore waist and an aching back, and insomnia. Although I had to take medicine and was examined frequently, the results were unsatisfactory. The doctors told me that I should not depend on medicine only but also take exercises. So I began to take exercises and mastered several practice methods.

Later, I went to the health qigong station, and learned the *Yi Jin Jing* Exercises, as well as *Ba Duan Jin*, *Liu Zi Jue* and *Wu Qin Xi*. I persist in practicing every morning. These four types of health qigong are easy to learn and understand. After practicing them, I feel comfortable and most of my bad feelings have disappeared. Now, I am clear-headed, have good eyesight, walk steadily, and seldom catch cold. This helps my children a lot, for they are not worried about taking care of me. Health qigong will become my closest companion during the last years of my life. Many neighbors have participated in practicing health qigong following me. Taking my own experience as an example, I'd like to spread the message about the merits of practicing health qigong.

Su Gui-ying
Hebei, China

When I began to learn Health Qigong—*Ba Duan Jin*, I imitated my instructor and bore his instructions carefully, such as "raise two arms with the center of the palms upward"; "raise the head and stare at the palms"; "shake the head and wag the back"; "squat slowly into the posture of Mabu chi"; "clench fists with open eyes" and so on. I was in a hurry to master them. However, just as the old saying, "more haste less speed", I was aching all over after three days' exercises, especially in my waist and arms. This made me be afraid of practicing health qigong.

After having rested at home for some time, I felt better and went to the health qigong station again. To my surprise, everyone had made great progress. Their actions were natural and they enjoyed doing it, especially when they did the action "waving the head and wagging the back". I suddenly realized that practicing *Ba Duan Jin* was not only for body building, but also for the enjoyment of the mind. So I began to practice it again.

This time I did not hurry to reach the goal but proceeded step by step. With the help of the instructor I tried my best to do the actions clearly and flexibly as well as to master the method of regulating the breathing. Gradually, I became used to doing it and many illnesses I have suffered for years, such as constipation and shoulder inflammation, have been cured.

Yi Si
Henan, China

When I first began to practice *Liu Zi Jue*, I thought as long as I could pronounce the sounds correctly with the right shape of the mouth I could master its essentials. So when I practiced, I focused on the standard action and the right shape of the mouth, and sometimes even used a mirror to correct myself. However, I couldn't stay relaxed while practicing, and there was little effect on my health. Later I realized that I had just imitated the actions mechanically without understanding the essentials of *Liu Zi Jue*.

In September 2004, with this problem, I took part in the lessons for health qigong instructors. After finishing the lesson, I knew that *Liu Zi Jue* emphasized the breathing assisted by the necessary action guiding, which demanded one should discharge the thick air-stream inside the body by regulating the breath to balance the circulation of the blood of the internal organs. But the premise is to stay relaxed in body and mind. Practitioners should banish distracting thoughts from their minds and concentrate on practicing to reach the realm of "calm, relaxed, peaceful, and concentrated" and stand up to the requirements of practicing health qigong. Get twice the result with half the effort.

Wang Jin-ping
Hebei, China

Appendix

Major Acupoints of the Human Body

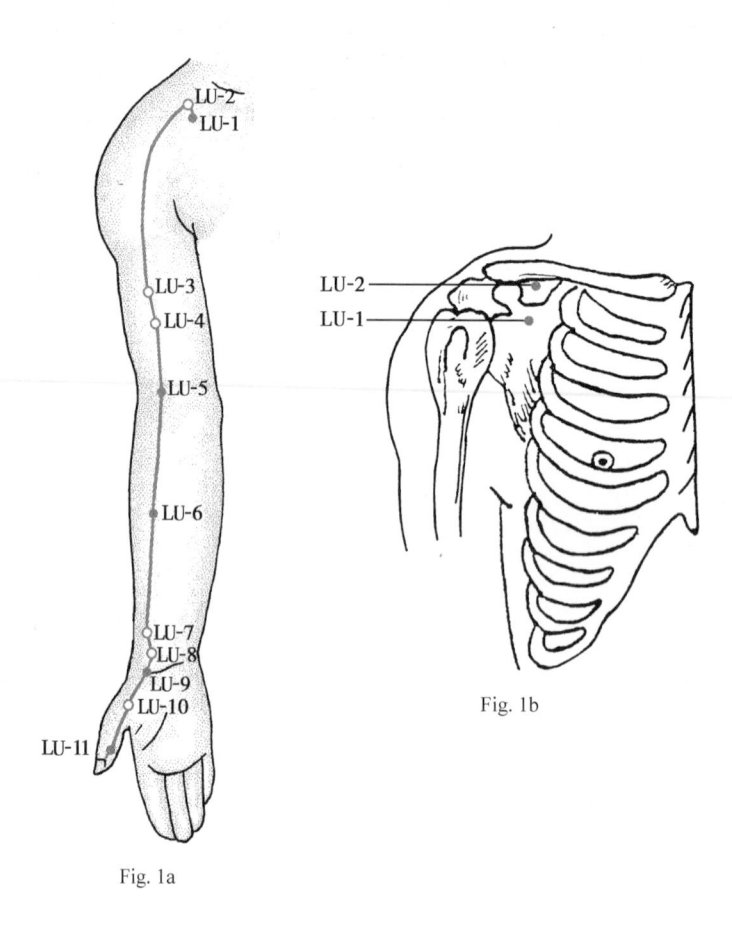

Fig. 1 Hand *taiyin* lung channel

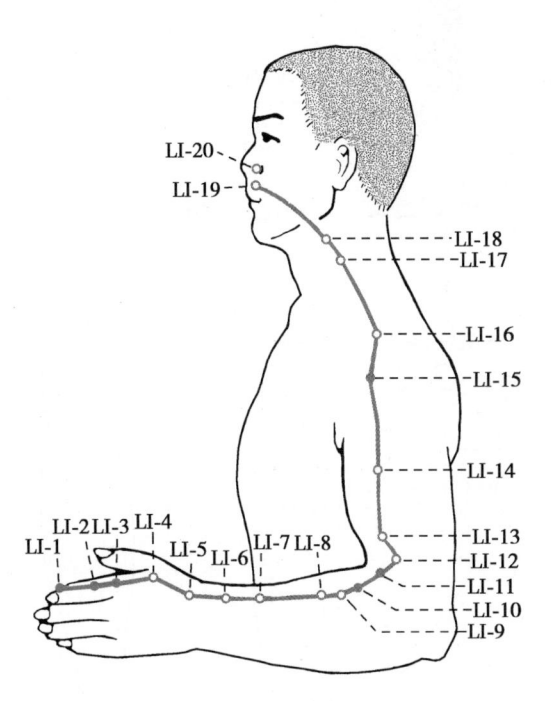

Fig. 2 Hand *yangming* large intestine channel

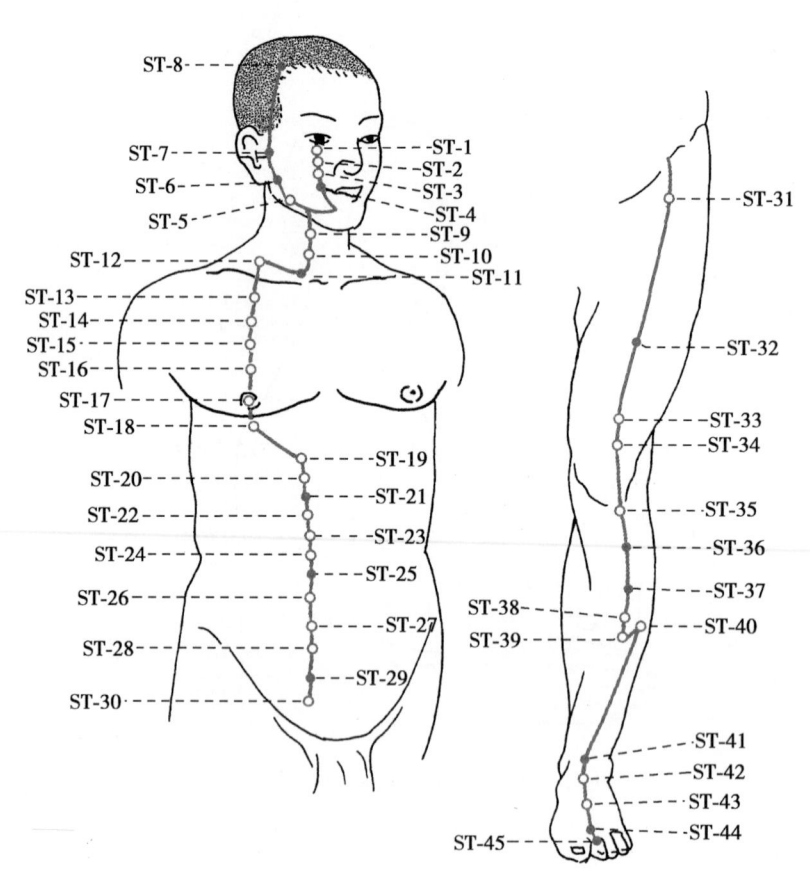

Fig. 3 Foot *yangming* stomach channel

Major Acupoints of the Human Body 129

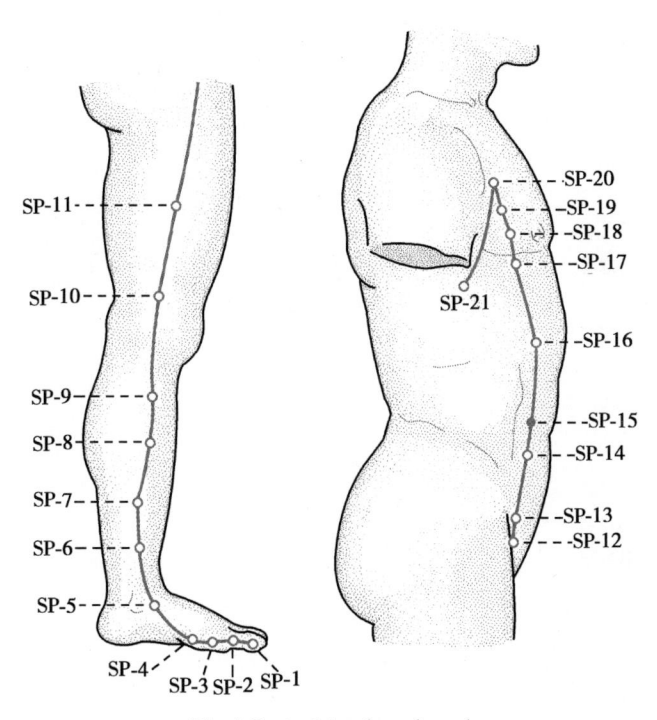

Fig. 4 Foot *taiyin* spleen channel

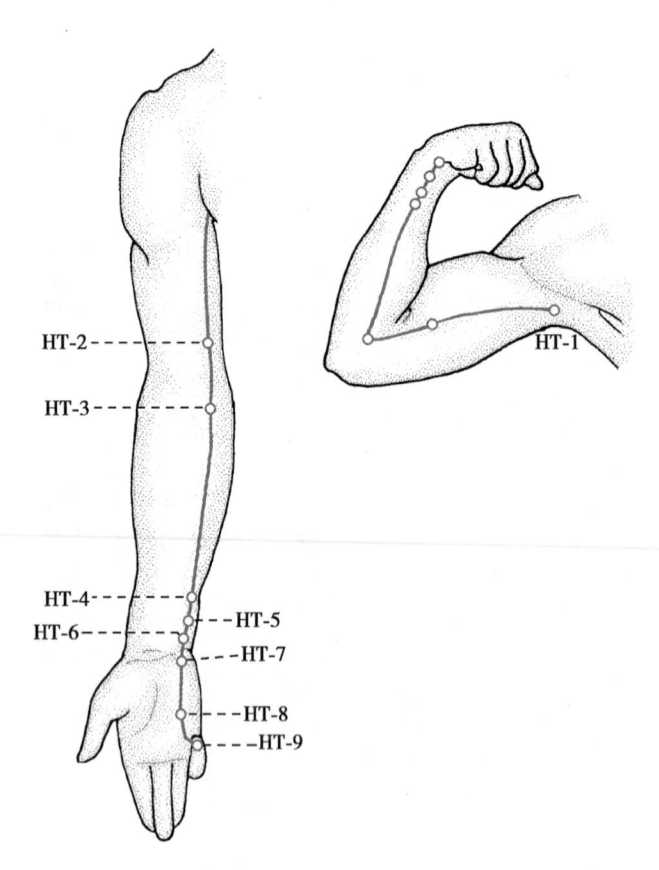

Fig. 5 Hand *shaoyin* heart channel

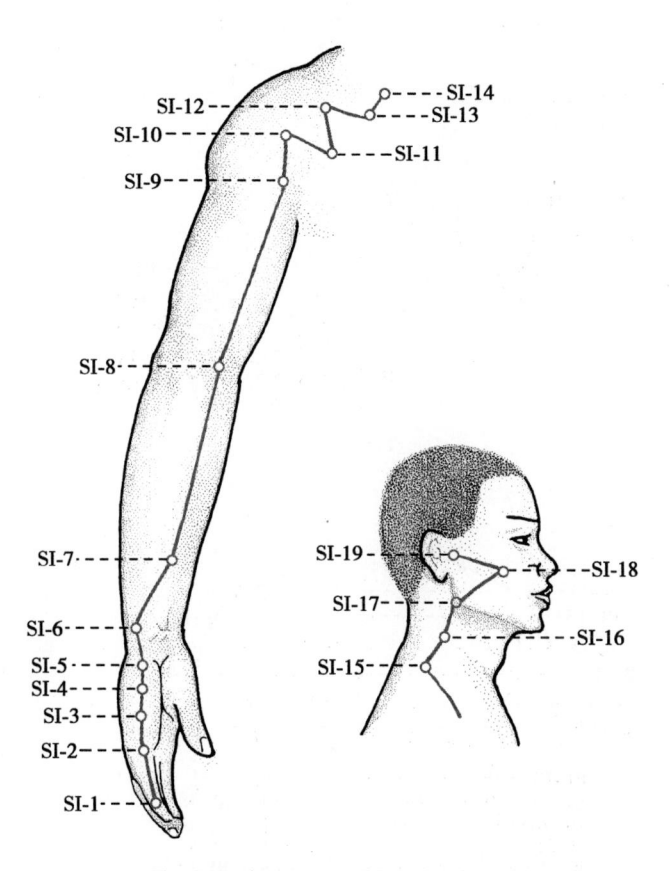

Fig. 6 Hand *taiyang* small intestine channel

Fig. 7a

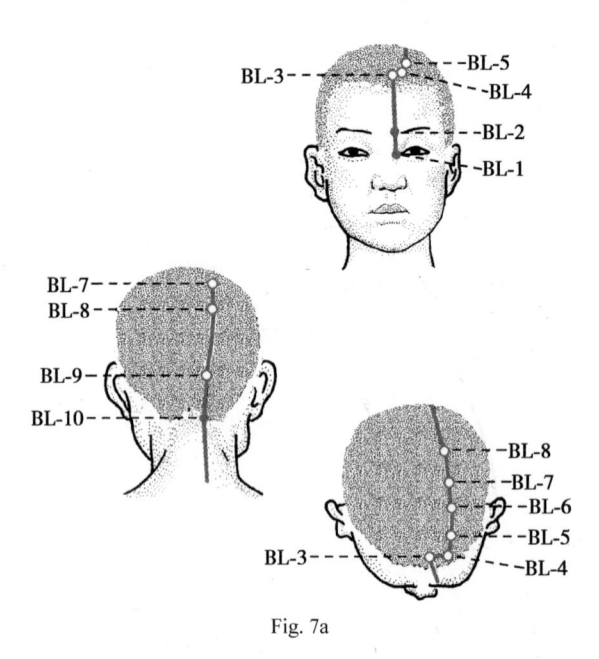

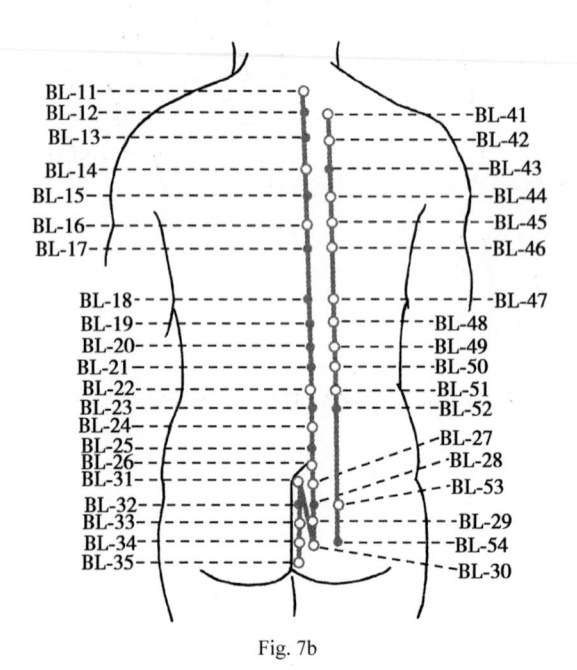

Fig. 7b

Major Acupoints of the Human Body 133

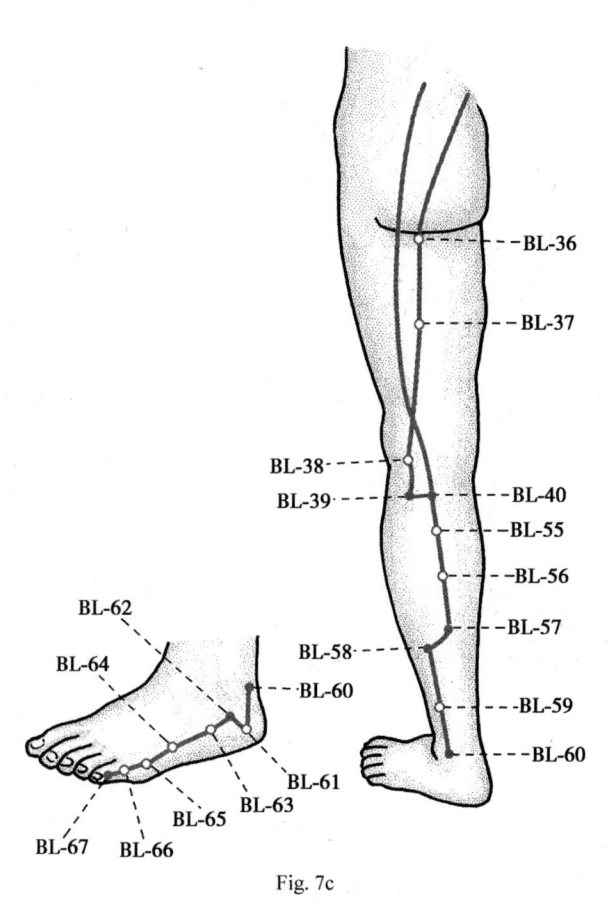

Fig. 7c

Fig. 7 Foot *taiyang* bladder channel

134 Appendix

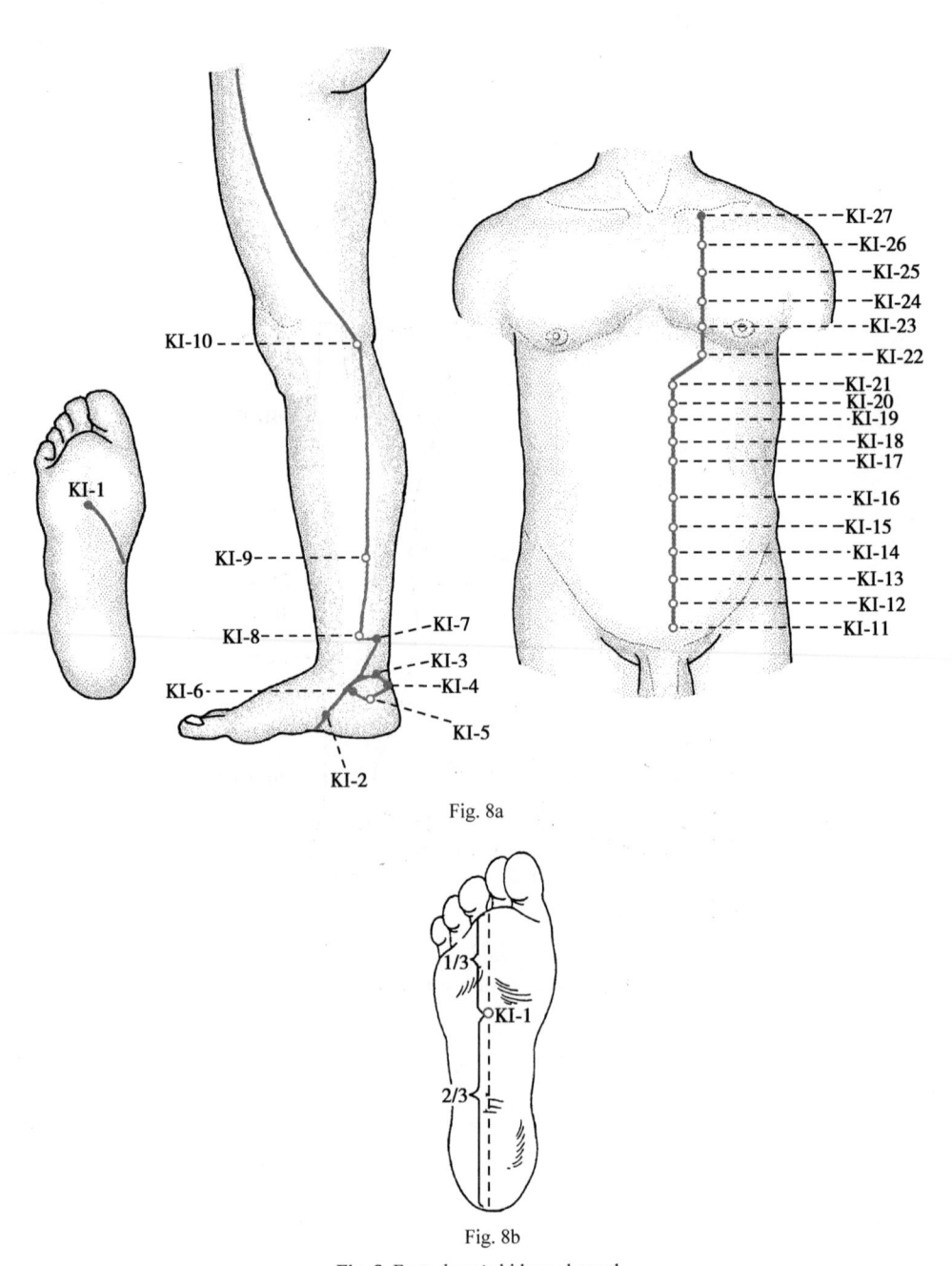

Fig. 8a

Fig. 8b

Fig. 8 Foot *shaoyin* kidney channel

Major Acupoints of the Human Body 135

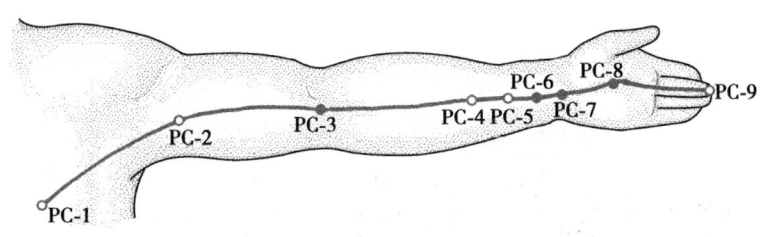

Fig. 9a

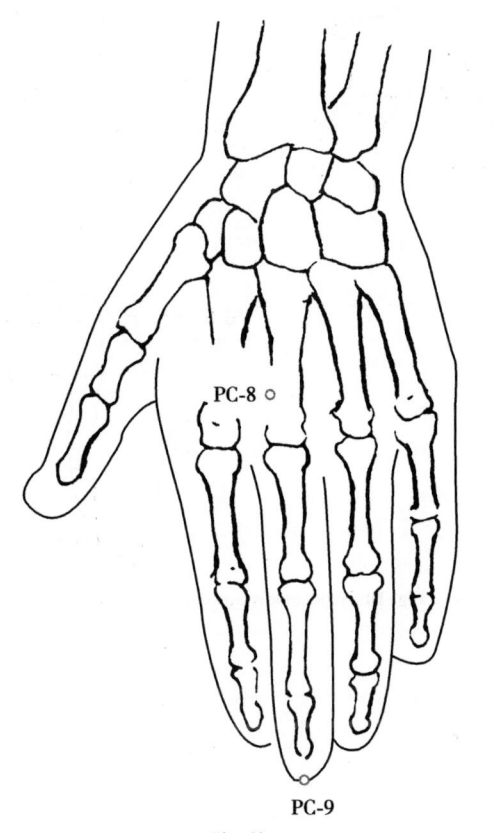

Fig. 9b

Fig. 9 Hand *jueyin* pericardium channel

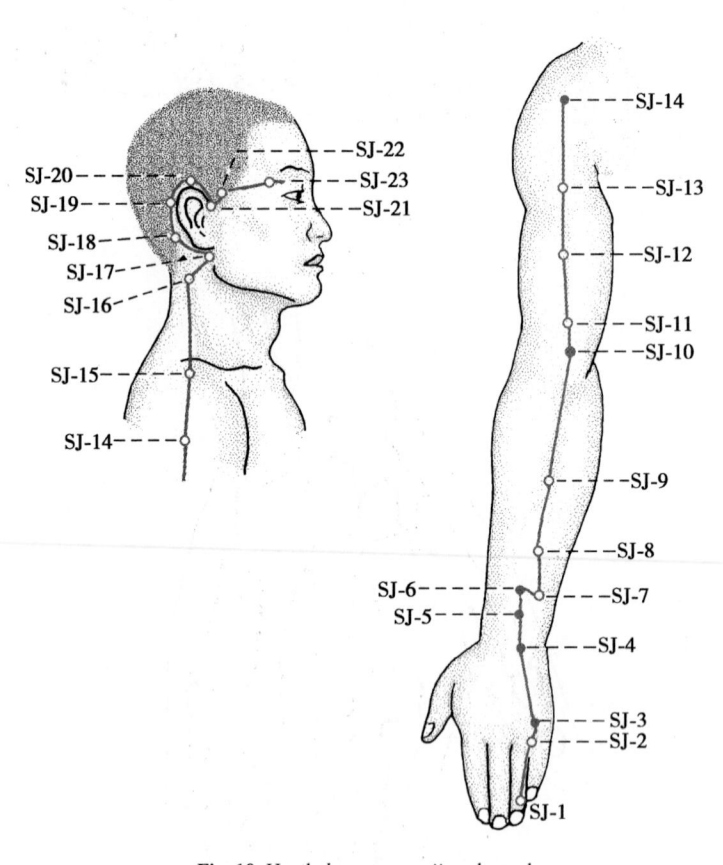

Fig. 10 Hand *shaoyang sanjiao* channel

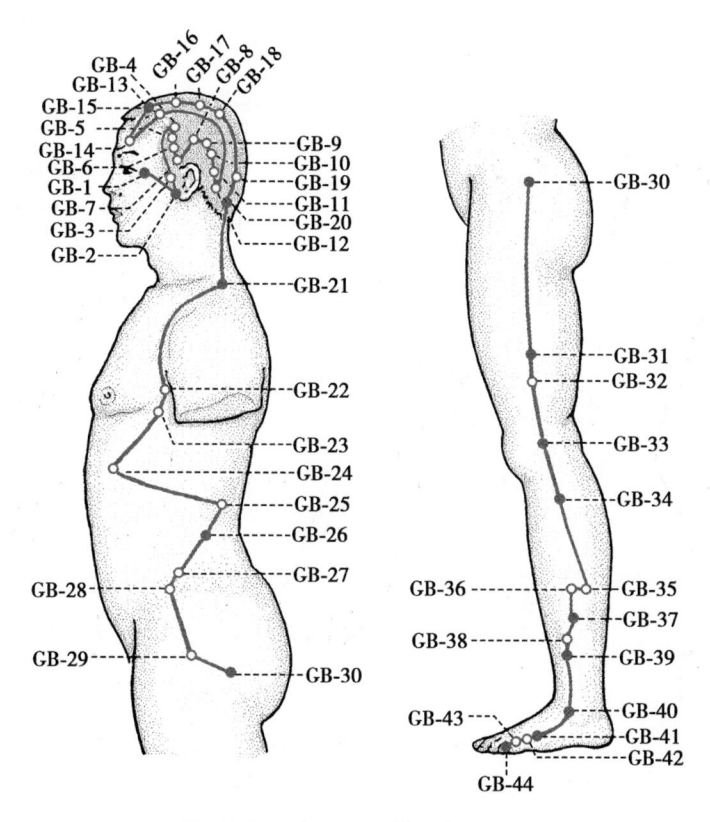

Fig. 11 Foot *shaoyang* gallbladder channel

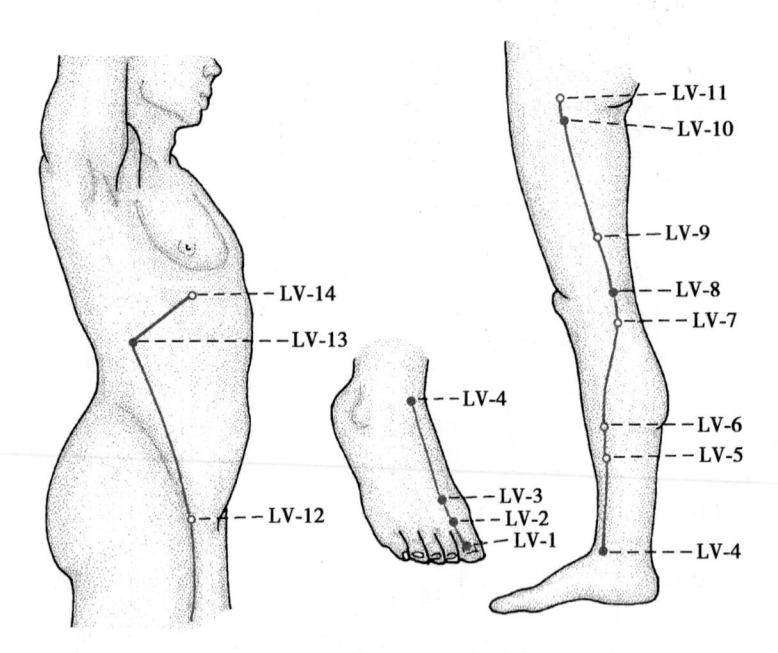

Fig. 12 Foot *jueyin* liver channel

Major Acupoints of the Human Body 139

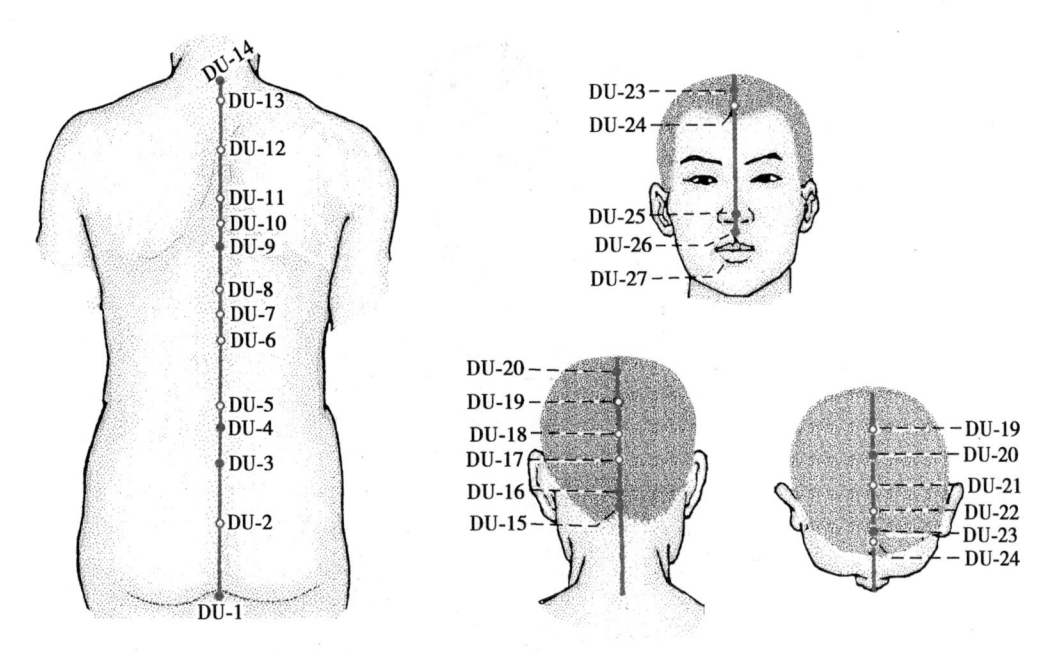

Fig. 13a

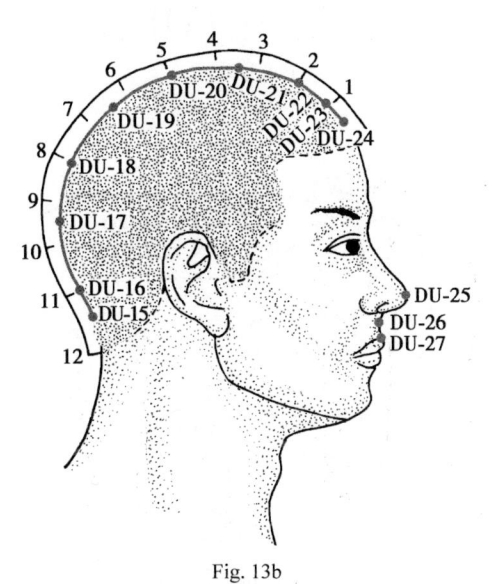

Fig. 13b

Fig. 13 *Du mai*

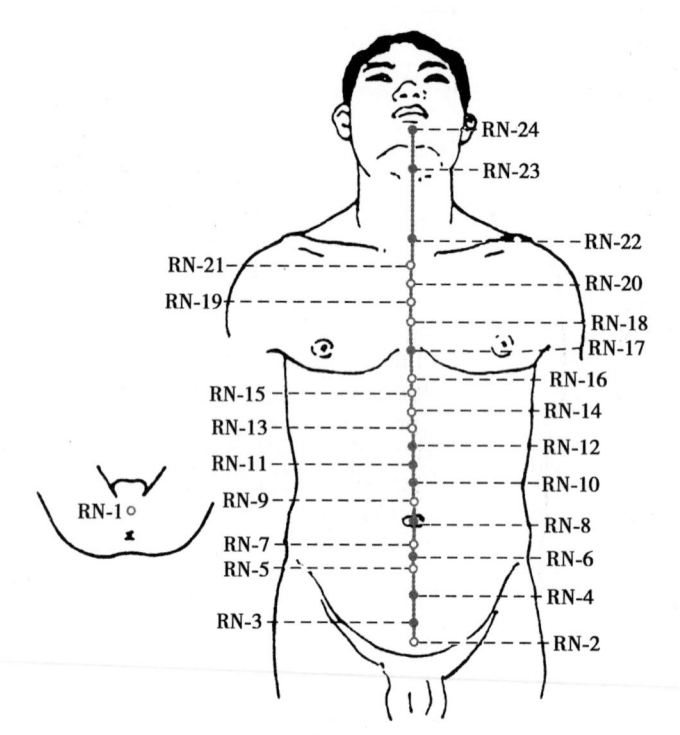

Fig. 14a

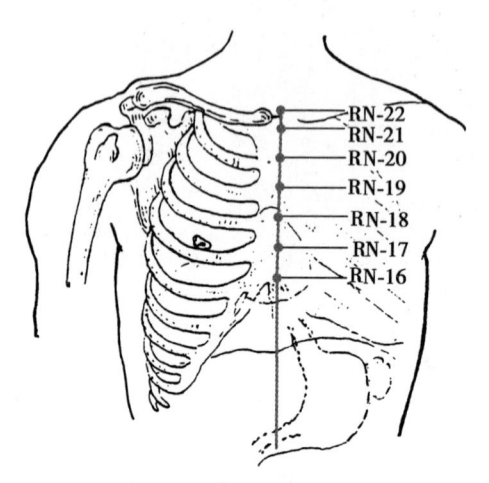

Fig. 14b

Fig. 14 *Ren mai*

Afterword

We are glad to bring this book to you. It is not an easy task to write and compile a qigong book that everyone can read and understand easily. The writers and editors of this book are mostly experts and scholars in health qigong study and health qigong teaching, but it is still a challenging mission for everyone. We sincerely pay our deep respects and appreciation to those who participated in this project. They showed great enthusiasm and passion for health qigong and contributed a lot to this book and to all practitioners of health qigong.

The main writers and editors who participated include (in alphabetical order):

- Cui Yong-sheng (Assistant Researcher, Health Qigong Management Center, China General Administration of Sports)
- Guo Shan-ru (Professor, Tianjin Institute of Technology)
- Hu Xiao-fei (Associate Professor, Beijing Sport University)
- Ke Xiao-jian (Lecturer, Hangzhou Teachers College – College of Sport and Health)
- Liu Yang (Research Trainee, Chinese Health Qigong Association)
- Song Tian-bin (Professor, Beijing University of Chinese Medicine)
- Xiang Han-ping (Associate Professor, Wuhan Institute of Physical Education)
- Yang Bai-long (Associate Professor, Beijing Sport University)
- Yu Ding-hai (Professor, Shanghai Institute of Physical Education)
- Zhang Jing (Associate Professor, Anqing Teachers College) & Wang Shu-ming (Professor, Anqing Teachers College)
- Zhang Ming-liang (Chinese Medicine Practitioner, Shanxi Huai-tang Acupuncture Institute)

In addition, Tao Zu-lai (Researcher, Institute of Mechanics, Chinese Academy of Sciences), Zhou Li-shang (Copy Editor, People's Sports Publishing House), Zhu Ying (Committee Member, Chinese Health Qigong Association), Song Tian-bin, Xiang Han-ping, and Zhang Ming-liang have contributed a lot to the structure of this book. Guo Shan-ru, Zhou Li-shang, and Song Tian-bin, Sun Fu-li (Researcher, XiYuan Hospital of China Academy of Traditional Chinese Medicine) have participated in the job of reviewing the drafts. Ji Yun-xi (Vice-Chairman, Chinese Health Qigong Association), and Zou Ji-jun (Vice-Chairman, Chinese Health Qigong Association) were responsible for organizing the drafts, with the help of Ding Dong (Deputy-Secretary-General, Chinese Health Qigong Association) and Cui Yong-sheng.

We apologize for failing to list all the references and quotes used in this book.

The *Health Qigong* magazine and Beijing Sport University Press gave us a lot of support and help in editing and publishing the original Chinese version of this book, and we would like to thank them as well.

This is our first attempt to explain the profound theories of health qigong by simple language, and there may be imperfections, so please feel free to contact us if you have any feedback or suggestions. We will work hard to continually improve in the future.

Editors
September 2010

Index

A
abdominal breathing, 15
alternative medicine, 5
arteriosclerosis, 51
atherosclerosis, 47
attention, 55

B
Ba Duan Jin, 35, 44, 50, 98, 119
bǎi huì, 27
BL 9, 85
blood pressure, 48
body regulation, 13, 24, 42, 90
breathing with anus-contracted, 15
breath regulation, 14, 50, 90

C
cerebrovascular diseases, 51
channels and collaterals, 18
chuī, 34, 96
Cun-xiang, 16

D
dān tián, 89
dàn zhōng, 89
daoyin diagram, 9
dietary health cultivation, 19
DU 20, 27
du mai, 100

E
EEG, 47
elixir field, 89
endocrine system, 47

F
Five Animals Frolic, 32

H
hē, 34, 94
health, 1
health cultivation, 75
health exercises, 5
health qigong, 12
hū, 34, 95

I
imagination, 56
immune system, 49
intelligence, 54
interpersonal relationships, 60

J
jiā jǐ, 85

K
KI 1, 27

L
láo gōng, 90
lifestyle, 21, 28
Liu Zi Jue, 34, 92, 118

M
medical health cultivation, 19
mental concentration, 16, 55
mental tranquility, 24
mind induction, 16
mind regulation, 27, 50, 58, 90

moderation, 2

N
nasal inhaling and mouth exhaling, 14
natural breathing, 14
nervous system, 47

P
PC 8, 90
personality, 58

Q
qi and blood, 24
qigong health cultivation, 18

R
Ready Position, 100, 103
RN 17, 89, 90

S
sī, 34, 95
Six Sounds, 34
sports prescriptions, 5
sub-health, 3

T
three regulations, 13, 58, 80
Traditional Chinese Health Cultivation (TCHC), 18
Traditional Chinese Medicine (TCM), 5
tranquility, 71
Type A personality, 59

W
Wu Qin Xi, 32, 49, 50, 88, 118

X
xī, 34, 97
xū, 34, 93

Y
Yi Jin Jing, 29, 44, 118
yin and yang, 24, 26, 27
Yi-shou, 16
yǒng quán, 27
yù zhěn, 85

图书在版编目（CIP）数据

走进健身气功=A Journey into Health Qigong：英文／中国健身气功协会主编．—北京：人民卫生出版社，2011.2
　　ISBN 978-7-117-13623-5

　Ⅰ.①走…　Ⅱ.①中…　Ⅲ.①气功－健身运动－英文　Ⅳ.①R214

中国版本图书馆CIP数据核字（2010）第210060号

门户网：www.pmph.com	出版物查询、网上书店
卫人网：www.ipmph.com	护士、医师、药师、中医师、卫生资格考试培训

走进健身气功（英文）

主　　编：中国健身气功协会
出版发行：人民卫生出版社（中继线 +8610-5978-7399）
地　　址：中国北京市朝阳区潘家园南里19号
　　　　　世界医药图书大厦B座
邮　　编：100021
网　　址：http://www.pmph.com
E－mail：pmph @ pmph.com
发　　行：pmphsales@gmail.com
购书热线：+8610-5978 7399/5978 7338（电话及传真）
开　　本：710×1000　1/16
版　　次：2011年2月第1版　2011年2月第1版第1次印刷
标准书号：ISBN 978-7-117-13623-5/R・13624

版权所有，侵权必究，打击盗版举报电话：+8610-5978-7482
（凡属印装质量问题请与本社销售中心联系退换）